PREVENTING
PROSTATE
CANCER

REDUCE YOUR RISK
WITH SIMPLE, PROACTIVE CHOICES

Benny Gavi, MD

Maya Eylon

Healthy Living Publications

Summertown, Tennessee

Library of Congress Cataloging-in-Publication Data available on request.

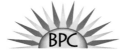

We chose to print this title on sustainably harvested paper stock certified by the Forest Stewardship Council®, an independent auditor of responsible forestry practices. For more information, visit us.fsc.org.

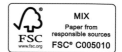

MIX
Paper from
responsible sources
FSC® C005010

Printed in the United States of America

Healthy Living Publications
an imprint of BPC
PO Box 99
Summertown, TN 38483
888-260-8458
bookpubco.com

ISBN: 978-1-57067-409-9

27 26 25 24 23 22   1 2 3 4 5 6 7 8 9

Contents

Preface

When I first started my internal medicine practice a decade ago, I met Mark. Mark was a new patient to my practice, but his congenial nature made him the type of man with whom you instantly connect. During our intake appointment, we were already comfortable talking freely, as if we had known each other for years. At first sight, Mark was your average American sixty-two-year-old man. He had a wonderful partner and two children in college. He had pronounced laugh lines around his mouth, and his eyes were a kind shade of brown. Having read Mark's medical records beforehand, I went into our first appointment also knowing that around a year ago he had successfully overcome prostate cancer.

When I broached the topic of his prostate cancer history during our appointment, the shift in his demeanor was palpable. At first he looked embarrassed, as if he was ashamed to talk about this terrible endeavor he had undergone. I couldn't help but wonder why. Surviving cancer is typically seen as a triumph of human nature and medical technology. Although it is a painful and arduous journey, I would have expected Mark to be proud, to some extent, of being a survivor, proud of defeating his cancerous enemy. Prior to this time, I did not have a notion of the true severity of prostate cancer. My education at Harvard Medical School had prepared me for the reality that men die from prostate cancer. My time as a hospital-based physician at Stanford had also made me aware of the fact that many men with prostate cancer would not die from their disease, because it is generally a slow-growing and often not aggressive disease. However, what I was not aware of was the number of possible long-term treatment side effects that many prostate cancer survivors live with.

Then Mark told me his story. I sat there, listening as this man opened up about the challenges he faced as a result of the life-saving, necessary therapies he had received to treat his prostate cancer. He did not look me in the eye as he talked about his struggles with urinary incontinence, the inability to control his urinary sphincter that resulted in him urinating when he did not want to. He averted his gaze when he discussed his difficulties dealing with sexual dysfunction. He talked about how this difficulty put a strain on his relationship with his wife. Not to mention that the strain on his relationship was only exacerbated by the financial and emotional burdens that accompanied his disease as well. His frustration was apparent as he spoke about the fatigue he experienced, a result of low testosterone.

I was at a loss for words. This man, who at first sight seemed happy and carefree, had been quietly dealing with the ongoing burdens of a disease that he wanted to move on from.

One of the most difficult parts of Mark's story was the realization that he is just one of the tens of thousands of men who silently suffer from prostate cancer and its aftermath. After this incredibly impactful appointment with Mark, I began researching prostate cancer. I read about how one in eight men in the United States are diagnosed with prostate cancer during their lifetime, an astoundingly high number for how little this disease is discussed. I read that although the mortality rate from this disease is significant, the difficult long-term effects on the survivors of this disease and its treatments are far more prevalent. That said, I also read that not all men experience long-term effects like the ones Mark struggled with, and for some the effects are temporary and can resolve with time. The more I read, the more I realized the lack of awareness of both the physical and emotional toll this disease has the potential to take on men. I became motivated to understand how this onerous condition could be prevented.

I read every article I could get my hands on about lifestyle factors and prostate cancer prevention, surprised by the magnitude of research that is currently available on the topic. It became clear that while newer surgical techniques, such as nerve sparing prostatectomies, and more advanced treatment options to improve testosterone levels and sexual health offer hope for men with prostate cancer today, there was a chance that I could help men reduce their risk for getting this disease in the first place, and perhaps even eliminate their risk altogether. I knew that if I could, it was my duty as a physician to provide all men with the knowledge they needed to decrease their chances of developing prostate cancer.

In 2019, I met Maya Eylon, an enthusiastic clinical researcher and medical student who was eager to study disease prevention. Together, with my vast medical knowledge and her research prowess, we became a powerful team, ready to tackle the masses of scientific literature on the prevention of prostate cancer through modifiable lifestyle factors.

And so our book was born.

For the past two years Maya and I have thoroughly reviewed hundreds of scientific studies on the connection between men's lifestyle choices and prostate cancer incidence. We created this book because we understand that you don't have the time to personally read all of these articles, but we believe you still deserve to have access to this information. You deserve to know the power of your choices and to make educated decisions when it comes to your health. We created this book to shed light on the burden of prostate cancer and hopefully improve the quality of life for men and their loved ones. We created the book for you: the physician, the nutritionist, the person hoping to prevent prostate cancer, the person recently diagnosed with prostate cancer, the loved one of someone with prostate cancer, and the individual who wants to learn more.

Our goal with this book wasn't to persuade you to live your life a certain way. Rather, our goal was to consolidate the masses of strong scientific data available today and present it to you in an accessible manner. This book reviews more than one hundred of the most recent, reliable, and relevant articles on the topic of lifestyle and prostate cancer. Each of these articles was deliberately selected, with as much objectivity as possible. We provide the data, so you can make informed decisions.

Prostate cancer is a serious disease that affects one in eight men in the United States. Current research indicates that you have the power to reduce your risk for prostate cancer incidence. Do not take our word for it; read this book and review the research yourself. Draw your own conclusions. Empower yourself.

Can You Prevent Prostate Cancer?

D oes the idea of having a prostate exam make you cringe? Do you feel your body tense up at the mere mention of the words? Doctors often recommend that men consider regularly testing for prostate cancer, and with good reason. Prostate cancer is the second most frequently diagnosed cancer in men around the world and the fifth leading cause of cancer deaths in men globally.[1] Within the United States specifically, the American Cancer Society (ACS) has found that one in eight men are diagnosed with prostate cancer within their lifetime and that one in forty-one men die from prostate cancer.[2] The average age for prostate cancer diagnosis in American men is sixty-five.

Prostate cancer occurs in the prostate, a walnut-sized gland that is located between the penis and the bladder, with the urethra running through its center. Prostates are responsible for producing the fluid that protects and transports sperm, also known as semen. Common treatments for prostate cancer include surgery, radiation, hormone therapy, and chemotherapy. The side effects from these treatments can

According to the American Cancer Society, 12.5% or 1 in 8 American men will be diagnosed with prostate cancer during their lifetime.

12.5%

significantly impact men's quality of life, and they range from urinary incontinence to erectile dysfunction, sepsis, and even death. While the mortality rate of prostate cancer is alarmingly high, the suffering that results from the symptoms and consequences of treating this disease are far more widespread. Millions of men quietly bear the effects of this terrible disease. You would be hard pressed to find an adult in the United States who has not in some way been personally impacted by this disease or, at the very least, knows someone who has been.

Yet, increasing knowledge of this disease has led to a shift in its perception over the years. The more the scientific and medical worlds learn about prostate cancer, the more portions of these communities are beginning to view this disease as preventable.[3]

You may now be asking yourself, "Preventable? How is that possible? Does this mean that the second most diagnosed cancer in American men could, to an extent, be avoided?" To answer these unsettling questions, let me tell you a series of stories that span decades of prostate cancer research and scientific discovery.

Fully understanding how prostate cancer became a topic of global interest starts with the publication of two international research studies that found one very shocking statistic. Over 70 percent of prostate cancer cases occur in developed countries.[1,4]

The first of these two studies was led by Ahmedin Jemal, DVM, PhD. Dr. Jemal is a recognized and well-respected researcher who has spent the past twenty years of his life working as a cancer epidemiologist for the American Cancer Society. Epidemiology is the part of medicine that works to understand why and where a disease occurs, how it spreads, and how we can control it. In one of his recent epidemiological studies, Dr. Jemal and his team of researchers worked with data from the World Health Organization to analyze the prostate cancer incidence and mortality rates in fifty-three countries around the world. He made several interesting discoveries.

Firstly, Dr. Jemal's findings showed that prostate cancer incidence rates have increased in thirty-two of the countries studied, with prostate cancer incidence rates being the highest in the countries with the most resources, such as the United States. In contrast, prostate cancer mortality rates have decreased in twenty-seven of the countries in the study. Generally, the decreased mortality rates were also observed in the countries that had more resources. The most shocking of Dr. Jemal's findings, though, was that over 70 percent of the prostate cancer cases analyzed in this study occurred in higher-resource, developed countries, such as New Zealand, countries in Western Europe, and the United States. Conversely, this meant that only 30 percent of prostate cancer cases occurred in lower-resource, developing countries, such as those in Southeast Asia and Northern Africa. This significant difference left Dr. Jemal wondering which factors could possibly be responsible for this disproportionate distribution of prostate cancer cases.

Initially, scientists believed the higher percentage of cases observed in developed countries was just the result of more cases being diagnosed. In other words, it wasn't that more men had prostate cancer in countries like the United States, but that the advanced medical technology used in these countries was detecting more cases.[4] While this theory was interesting, it lost traction once scientists found that there was already a fifty-fold difference in prostate cancer rates between countries before advanced testing technology was even created.[4] Furthermore, the authors of this study found that as countries around the world developed, their rates of prostate cancer increased, regardless of their diagnostic techniques.[1]

If advanced technology could not entirely account for this huge difference in incidence rates between countries, what could? Let's look a little deeper into this global study. Dr. Jemal's findings showed that while incidence rates were very high in the United States, they were relatively low in certain parts of Asia.[1–4] For example, compared to the alarming 213,700 new prostate cancer cases found in North America in 2008, fewer than 20,000 cases were recorded in Southeast Asia that same year.[4] When adjusted for population size, that means that twenty times more prostate cancer cases were recorded in North America than in Southeast Asia.

North America and South-Central Asia have an even more drastic difference, with nearly fifty times more cases of prostate cancer reported in North America than in South-Central Asia.[4]

It is one thing to read about the huge differences in incidence rates between countries, but it is another thing to see these differences with your own eyes. The graph below was adopted from the 2018 Global Cancer Statistics (GLOBOCAN). GLOBOCAN is a large-scale study that analyzes data from 185 countries and thirty-six different types of cancers to determine the most up-to-date estimations of worldwide cancer incidence and mortality. Look at the uneven distribution in this graph. Regions at the top of the graph (like Australia/New Zealand, Northern Europe, and North America) have incredibly higher reported rates of prostate cancer when compared to the countries at the bottom (like Northern Africa and South-Central Asia). This graph

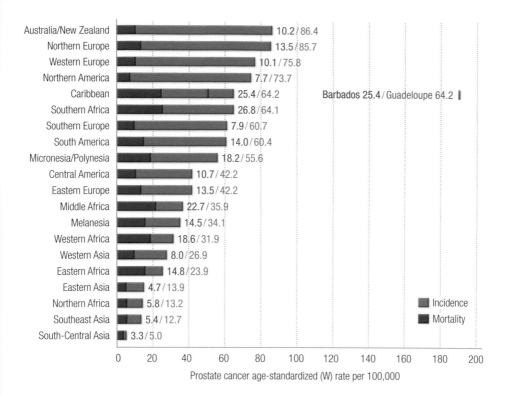

Prostate cancer age-standardized (W) rate per 100,000

shows the vast difference in prostate cancer rates by location, in a way that words cannot describe.

How could it be that the United States' second most diagnosed cancer is seemingly rare in parts of Asia? After this data was revealed, scientists from the University of Hawaii and the University of Southern California began exploring the role of ethnicity in prostate cancer incidence. They hypothesized that perhaps the huge difference in prostate cancer rates between countries was due to differences in ethnicity. For their study, these scientists looked at more than 215,000 study participants of varying socioeconomic status and ethnic identity to determine if ethnicity does in fact have an impact on prostate cancer incidence.[5] Specifically, they looked at Japanese men who had migrated from Japan, a country with low rates of prostate cancer, to the United States, a country with one of the highest rates of prostate cancer. What they discovered was extraordinary.

After analysis, these researchers found that prostate cancer risk in participants within the same ethnic group was reflective of the incidence rates in their country of residence, not their country of origin. The study participants who had migrated from countries with low prostate incidence (such as Japan) to areas of high incidence (such as America) displayed drastic increases in their rates of prostate cancer occurrence post-migration. Specifically, these researchers observed that within one generation of migration, after only four years of living in the United States, the Japanese study participants showed a 700 percent increase in their prostate cancer incidence rates. Shockingly, this increased incidence rate is still only half that seen in Caucasian Americans.[5]

Maybe this massive increase only occurred because we test for prostate cancer more frequently in the United States? The thing is, prostate cancer wasn't the only cancer to display a drastic shift in incidence in the individuals in this research study. The graph below, cropped from the original study, shows that the rate of stomach cancer in this Japanese migrant population was cut in half after one generation post-migration.[5] Like prostate cancer, breast cancer rates shot up. This graph shows that the overall shift in cancer rates may not be the result of more testing because we see some cancers decrease in incidence and other cancers increase.[5]

A second study continued this research by looking at the relative roles of environment, genetics, and ethnicity in incidence and mortality rates of prostate cancer.[6] The study's results showed that Chinese Americans and Japanese Americans had significantly higher rates of incidence and mortality from prostate cancer when compared to individuals of their same ethnicity still living in China and Japan,

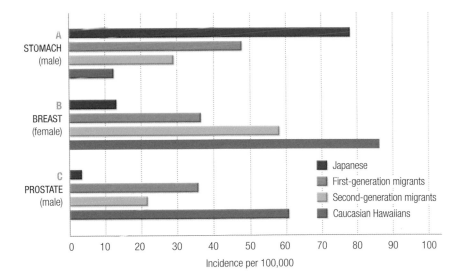

respectively. In fact, these scientists found that Chinese study participants living in America had sixteen times more prostate cancer incidences than the Chinese participants living in China.[6]

Based on these findings, it does not appear that ethnicity was what protected the men in these studies from prostate cancer because, in both cases, after the participants began living in the United States their incidence rates skyrocketed.

With the help of these scientific studies, we now have the understanding that ethnicity and cancer testing technology may play a smaller role in your prostate cancer risk than scientists previously believed, but what about genetics? How much of your prostate cancer risk is heritable, meaning it is transferred down to you from family members through your genes? Another way to look at heritability when it comes to cancer incidence is the portion of a population's cancer variation that can be attributed to individual genetic differences.

To answer this epidemiological question, we will look at two of the most reputable twin studies on this exact topic. But, before we discuss these studies, let's talk about why we look at twin studies to answer questions about diseases and genetics. Put simply, twin studies are the best way to understand the heritability of a disease because identical twins have the same genetic codes. Therefore, they provide a unique perspective for observing the role of nature (genetics) versus nurture (environment) in determining the root cause(s) of a disease. The basic idea of these studies is that if a disease is heritable it's most likely that either both twins will get the same disease or both won't. On the flip side, if the disease is not as heavily based on genetics, in some cases one twin could get the disease and the other won't.

Paul Lichtenstein, Dr. Med., a professor of genetic epidemiology, has dedicated his life thus far to understanding the role of genetics in human health. Dr. Lichtenstein has unique insight into the power of twin studies as the former head of the largest twin registry in the world, the Swedish Twin Registry (STR). Harnessing the power of the STR, Dr. Lichtenstein and his colleagues conducted a study to deter-

42%   How much of prostate cancer risk is heritable? According to research conducted by Dr. Lichtenstein and his colleagues, 42% of your risk is related to your genes 58% of your risk is unrelated to your genes.   **58%**

mine how much of prostate cancer risk is heritable.[7] Looking at data from 89,576 twin individuals, this study found that heritability was a statistically significant risk factor for prostate cancer. Specifically, the results showed that 42 percent of the study participants' prostate cancer risk could be attributed to their genetics[7]. Breaking down this statistic and applying it to your life, this means that approximately 42 percent of your risk for getting prostate cancer could be due to genetics. While 42 percent is no doubt a weighty percentage, this statistic also implies that nearly 60 percent of your risk is entirely unrelated to your genes. Based on his findings, Dr. Lichtenstein suggested that a man's environment could be the primary contributor to his prostate cancer risk, not genetics.[7] So even if your father or grandfather had prostate cancer, your fate isn't necessarily sealed, because more than half of your risk for this disease falls outside of your genes.

If you are unsatisfied with Dr. Lichtenstein's study alone, a second, more extensive twin study exists. In this next study researchers looked at data from 203,691 twin individuals in the Nordic Twin Study of Cancer (NorTwinCan) to assess the relative impact of genetics versus environment in prostate cancer incidence.[8] After following their study subjects for more than three decades, the researchers in this study found that heritability accounted for 57 percent of the observed prostate cancer cases. Unlike Dr. Lichtenstein's findings, these results imply that the primary cause of prostate cancer incidence is heritability.[8] Similarly to Dr. Lichtenstein's findings, these results also imply that genetics don't explain all of your risk for this disease. In this study, 43 percent of risk cannot be attributed to heritability, meaning environmental factors do still play a big role in your risk for prostate cancer.[8] These researchers recognized this fact as well, which is why, despite its relatively high level of heritability, they chose to still emphasize the importance of environment, lifestyle factors, and preventive measures in prostate cancer risk and incidence at the end of their article.

One by one, researchers around the world have shifted toward a new understanding of the environment as a major contributor to men's individual risk for prostate cancer incidence. A central component of an individual's environment are their lifestyle choices.[1-11]

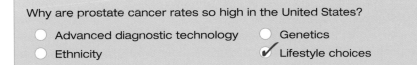

Why are prostate cancer rates so high in the United States?

- ○ Advanced diagnostic technology
- ○ Ethnicity
- ○ Genetics
- ✓ Lifestyle choices

Lifestyle choices are the daily practices we have, from our diets to our exercising patterns. After three decades of research, scientists today believe that the seemingly small decisions we make every day may be the key to preventing prostate cancer.

Wait one minute. Let's be honest: Just how much of an effect could eating an extra daily serving of veggies have on your risk of getting prostate cancer?

47%

Based on study findings, Dr. Stacey Kenfield and colleagues estimate that 47% of terminal prostate cancer cases in America can be prevented through healthier lifestyle choices.

Stacey Kenfield, ScD, and her colleagues in California asked this same question when conducting a study to quantify the impact of everyday lifestyle choices in prostate cancer risk and incidence.[9] For her study, Dr. Kenfield harnessed thirty years' worth of data from 42,701 men in the Health Professionals Follow-Up Study and 20,324 men in the Physicians' Health Study. The lifestyle information Dr. Kenfield collected from these men centered on daily practices and general bodily measurements, including diet, physical activity, body mass index (BMI), and smoking habits. No one could have predicted the staggering results Dr. Kenfield would find. Of the men studied, results showed that those who followed the healthiest lifestyle practices had a 68 percent decrease in terminal prostate cancer incidence when compared to the men who had the least healthy lifestyles. In other words, by simply adhering to healthier life choices, these men were able to effectively reduce their risk of dying from prostate cancer by an astounding 68 percent.[9] What's more, based on her findings Dr. Kenfield predicted that nearly half of the deadly prostate cancer cases in the United States could be prevented if men followed a healthier lifestyle.[9]

Like the men in Dr. Kenfield's study, you too have the power to make healthier choices to reduce your risk of getting prostate cancer. While things like genetics are out of your control, research has shown that there are real, tangible ways to reduce your risk for prostate cancer that are within your control. Over the course of this book, we will review the specific healthy lifestyle choices, from diet to exercise, that you can integrate into your daily practices to help prevent prostate cancer.

While these scientists may have found that lifestyle choices have an unparalleled impact on reducing prostate cancer risk, this is just one study, so it's understandable if you are still skeptical. Here's the thing: this study is not alone. The American Cancer Society stated in their latest guidelines for cancer prevention that "most of the variation in cancer risk across populations and among individuals is due to factors that are not inherited."[10] The ACS is saying that the major causes of differences in prostate cancer risk and incidence between people are not unchangeable factors like our genes, but instead are the choices we make in our everyday lives.

Now that we have established that a healthy lifestyle can make all the difference in your risk for prostate cancer, you may be asking yourself, "What is a healthy lifestyle?" Once again, the ACS can help us out. Every few years the ACS compiles all of the current research on lifestyle practices and cancer to create a comprehensive set of recommendations for how Americans can live a cancer-preventing lifestyle. In their guidelines, the ACS makes evidence- and research-based suggestions on both the healthful practices that you should increase and unhealthy practices you should decrease. Within these recommendations, the ACS highlights diet, physical activity, and body weight as the most important risk factors to focus on when working toward reducing your prostate cancer risk.[10] The great thing about these factors is that they are modifiable, which means that you have the power to turn all three into preventative measures against prostate cancer, just by making healthy choices in your daily life. When it comes to diet, your goal should be to eat nutrient-filled foods, such as whole grains, soy products, beans, and at least two and a half cups of colorful vegetables every day.[10] In addition to the healthy foods you should eat, avoid consuming most animal products, especially red meat, eggs, and dairy products. In regard to physical activity, your key to success is dedicating at least 150 minutes per week to exercise. That's only

1 DIET	2 EXERCISE	3 REMEMBER
2½ cups of vegetables per day, whole grains, soy products, beans	150 minutes per week of physical activity	Limit your intake of alcohol and stop smoking completely
Avoid most animal products, especially beef, eggs, milk	(That's only 20 minutes per day!)	

20 minutes per day! Finally, an important part of a healthy lifestyle is limiting alcohol intake and eliminating any smoking habits.[10] In the following chapters, we will delve into the specific benefits of implementing these healthy practices into your day-to-day lives.

Looking at this long list of lifestyle changes can be overwhelming. There may be a part of you that is now thinking, "What is the point of trying if I can't make all of these changes?" Your goal should not be to change your entire life overnight, but rather to take small steps in the right direction. Scientists recognize that sometimes we need a little push to get started on the right path, so several researchers in Sweden conducted a research experiment to determine the effects of a single hour of exercise on men's ability to fight prostate cancer.[11]

In this experiment, the researchers took blood samples from men before they exercised and then compared these pre-exercise samples to samples drawn after the men exercised intensively for only sixty-five minutes. In this way, each participant in this study acted as their own baseline control. Prostate cancer cells (LNCaP) were then added to both the pre- and post-exercise blood samples and the results were recorded. Findings showed that after exercising, the men's blood naturally fought off the prostate cancer cells 31 percent more effectively than their blood before exercising.[11] If just one hour of exercise made such a significant difference in these men's ability to destroy cancer cells, imagine what two hours could do.

Arguably, the best part about making healthier lifestyle choices is the "double-dipping" nature of these changes. Not only does a healthy lifestyle reduce your risk for one of America's most frequently diagnosed cancers, but it can also reduce your risk for our nation's other leading causes of death.[12–15] Let's start by looking at the top causes of mortality in the United States. In 2018, the Centers for Disease Control

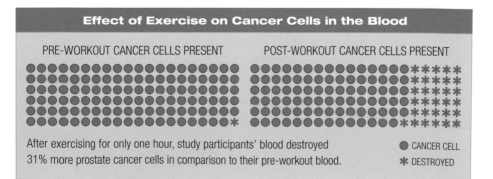

Effect of Exercise on Cancer Cells in the Blood

PRE-WORKOUT CANCER CELLS PRESENT   POST-WORKOUT CANCER CELLS PRESENT

After exercising for only one hour, study participants' blood destroyed 31% more prostate cancer cells in comparison to their pre-workout blood.

● CANCER CELL
✱ DESTROYED

(CDC) published a report on this exact topic. Included in this report is a breakdown of the ten leading causes of death in the United States. In death toll order these killers are heart disease, cancer, unintentional injury, chronic lower respiratory disease, stroke, Alzheimer's disease, diabetes, influenza and pneumonia, suicide, and kidney disease. Data for this report was drawn from the death certificates filed in all fifty states and the District of Columbia in 2016 and 2017. The graph below is a summary of the top ten causes of death in the United States and their relative death tolls in 2016 and 2017.[12]

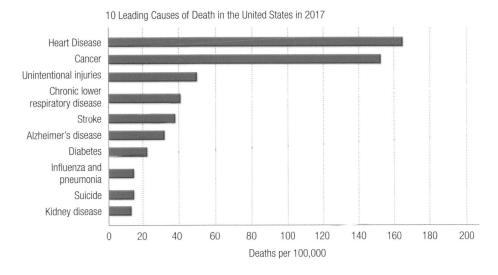

In the spirit of keeping things short and to the point, we will only explore the double-dipping health benefits of lifestyle changes in reducing your risk for a few of the United States' top killers, starting with our number one killer: heart disease.

In 2004, a global study was conducted with data from fifty-two countries to see if lifestyle impacted people's risk for acute myocardial infarctions, also known as heart attacks.[13] This study, led by Salim Yusuf, MD, an internationally recognized cardiologist, analyzed data from 12,461 recorded cases of myocardial infarction and 14,637 controls. Specifically, the goal of this study was to evaluate the role of nine lifestyle practices in causing heart attacks. Seven of the nine factors were considered to be "risk factors" for getting a heart attack: smoking, drinking, abnormal lipids, psychosocial factors, hypertension, diabetes, and obesity. The other two factors were considered to be protective against heart attacks: eating fruits and vegetables, and physical activity. After analysis, these researchers found that the same lifestyle choices that reduce your risk for prostate cancer (diet and physical activity) can also reduce your risk for heart attacks. In fact, the researchers determined that the total impact of these lifestyle factors accounted for over 90 percent of participants' risk for initial heart attacks. Furthermore, they found that by altering these factors, participants had the potential to prevent future heart attacks. These significant results were also seen when looking at people's risks for stroke (fifth leading killer in America) and type 2 diabetes (seventh leading killer in America).[14, 15]

By making simple, healthy lifestyle changes, you not only reduce your risk for prostate cancer but also protect yourself against the other leading causes of death in the United States.

Current research indicates that your risk of prostate cancer can be reduced, and even prevented. You have the power to possibly prevent prostate cancer and this power comes in the form of daily lifestyle choices. Ask more questions. Talk to your doctor. Become engaged in your health. You might assume that if something was important to your health, your doctor would mention it. Unfortunately, your health is too valuable to wait for medical professionals to have all the answers.

Throughout this book we will discuss the major healthy practices that you can integrate into your life to decrease your risk for getting prostate cancer. In the coming pages you will learn about prostate health superfoods, like broccoli and soy, as well as potentially harmful foods to avoid for a healthier, cancer-preventing lifestyle. You will review powerful data on obesity and the benefits of exercise in reducing your risk for prostate cancer. Finally, you will learn about the various routine prostate cancer–screening options available today and how these options relate to you.

Read on. Use this information to take ownership over your health. There is no time like the present.

BIBLIOGRAPHY CHAPTER 1

1. Bray, F., Ferlay, J., Soerjomataram, I., Siegel, R.L., Torre, L.A., and Jemal, A. (2018). Global cancer statistics 2018: GLOBOCAN estimates of incidence and mortality worldwide for 36 cancers in 185 countries. *CA: A Cancer Journal for Clinicians*, 68(6):394–424. DOI:10.8822/caac.21492.

2. The American Cancer Society Medical and Editorial Content Team. "Key Statistics for Prostate Cancer." Accessed January 8, 2020. www.cancer.org/cancer/prostate-cancer/about/key-statistics.html.

3. Chan, R., Lok, K., and Woo, J. (2009). Prostate cancer and vegetable consumption. *Molecular Nutrition and Food Research*, 53(2):201–216. DOI:10.1002/mnfr.200800113.

4. Center, M.M., Jemal, A., Lortet-Tieulent, J., Ward, E., Ferlay, J., Brawley, O., and Bray, F. (2012). International variation in prostate cancer incidence and mortality rates. *European Urology*, 61(6):1079–1092. DOI:10.1016/j.eururo.2012.02.054.

5. Kolonel, L.N., Altshuler, D., and Henderson, E. (2004). The multiethnic cohort study exploring genes, lifestyle and cancer risk. *Nature Reviews Cancer*, 4(7):519–527. DOI:10.1038/nrc1389.

6. Hsing, A.W., Tsao, L., and Devesa, S.S. (2000). International trends and patterns of prostate cancer incidence and mortality. *International Journal of Cancer*, 85(1):60–67. DOI:10.1002/(sici)1097-0215(20000101)85:1<60::aid-ijc11>3.0.co:2-b.

7. Lichtenstein, P., Holm, N.V., Verkasalo, P.K., Iliadou, A., Kaprio, J., Koskenvuo, M., Pukkala, E., et al. (2000). Environmental and heritable factors in the causation of cancer—analyses of cohorts of twins from Sweden, Denmark, and Finland. *The New England Journal of Medicine*, 343(2):78–85. DOI:10.1056/NEJM200007133430201.

8. Mucci, L.A., Hjelmborg, J.B., Harris, J.R., Czene, K., Havelick, D.J., Scheike, T., Graff, R.E., et al. (2016). Familial risk and heritability of cancer among twins in Nordic countries. *JAMA*, 315(1):68–76. DOI:10.1001/jama.2015.17703.

9. Kenfield, S.A., Batista, J.L., Jahn, J.L., Downer, M.K., Van Blarigan, E.L., Sesso, H.D., Giovannucci, E.L., et al. (2015). Development and application of a lifestyle score for prevention of lethal prostate cancer. *Journal of the National Cancer Institute*, 108(3), djv329. DOI: 10.1093/jnci/djv329.

10. Kushi, L.H., Doyle, C., McCullough, M., Rock, C.L., Demark-Wahnefried, W., Bandera, E.V., Gapstur, S., et al. (2012). American Cancer Society guidelines on nutrition and physical activity for cancer prevention: reducing the risk of cancer with healthy food choices and physical activity. *CA: A Cancer Journal for Clinicians*, 62(1):30–67. DOI:10.3322/caac.20140.

11. Rundqvist, H., Augsten, M., Strömberg, A., Rullman, E., Mijwel, S., Kharaziha, P., Panaretakis, T., et al. (2013). Effect of acute exercise on prostate cancer cell growth. *PLoS One*, 8(7):e67579. DOI:10.1371/journal.pone.0067579.

12. Murphy, S.L., Xu, J.Q., Kochanek, K.D., Arias, E. (2018). "Mortality in the United States, 2017." *NCHS Data Brief*, no 328. National Center for Health Statistics. www.cdc.gov/nchs/products/databriefs/db328.htm.

13. Yusuf, S., Hawken, S., Ounpuu, S., Dans, T., Avezum, A., Lanas, F., McQueen, M., et al. (2004). Effect of potentially modifiable risk factors associated with myocardial infarction in 52 countries (the INTERHEART study): case-control study. *Lancet*, 364(9438):937–952. DOI:10.1016/S0140-6736(04)17018-9.

Additional Studies Not Detailed in the Chapter

14. Chiuve, S.E., Rexrode, K.M., Spiegelman, D., Logroscino, G., Manson, J.E., and Rimm, E.B. (2008). Primary prevention of stroke by healthy lifestyle. *Circulation*, 118(9):947–954. DOI:10.1161/CIRCULATIONAHA.108.781062.

     Following more than 100,000 subjects (43,685 men from the Health Professionals Follow-up Study and 71,243 women from the Nurses' Health Study), this study aimed to determine the impact of lifestyle on stroke risk. A low-risk lifestyle, as defined by the study, included not smoking, a BMI under 25 kg/m^2, exercising for at least thirty minutes per day, limited consumption of alcohol, and scoring in the top 40 percent of a healthy diet score. Findings indicated that up to 54 percent of strokes in women and 52 percent of strokes in men can potentially be prevented through healthy lifestyle practices.

15. Tuomilehto, J., Lindström, J., Eriksson, J.G., Valle, T.T., Hämäläinen, H., Ilanne-Parikka, P., Keinänen-Kiukaanniemi, S., et al. (2001). Prevention of type 2 diabetes mellitus by changes in lifestyle among subjects with impaired glucose tolerance. *The New England Journal of Medicine*, 344(18):1343–1350. DOI:10.1056/NEJM200105033441801.

     With the goal of preventing type 2 diabetes, researchers in Finland created and evaluated the effects of a lifestyle intervention program on subjects who were at high risk for developing type 2 diabetes. The intervention program included individualized counseling for weight reduction, dietary alterations, and increasing physical activity. The study consisted of 522 overweight subjects with impaired glucose tolerance, who were randomly assigned to either the intervention group or control group. Results showed that over the course of the study, the subjects in the intervention group, when compared to the control group, reduced their risk for type 2 diabetes by 58 percent. This significant reduction in risk was found to be directly associated with the intervention program's lifestyle changes.

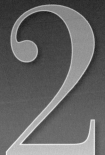

CHAPTER

Vegetables and Cruciferous Vegetables

2

he way you choose to nourish your body is a decision you make every day. A decision that, whether or not you realize it, gives you the power to prevent diseases. When it comes to your diet, small choices can make a big impact on your health. Current research on the topic of nutrition, dietary practices, and prostate cancer prevention has all led to the same conclusion: eating more vegetables can help reduce your risk for prostate cancer.[1-5] In this chapter we will not only discuss the impact of overall vegetable intake on your risk for prostate cancer but also explore a veggie subgroup known as cruciferous vegetables and their unique anti-cancer properties.

Unlike the warnings your doctor will undoubtedly give you about the possible dangers associated with the medical treatments for prostate cancer, you won't find many doctors who will warn you against the dangers of eating broccoli. There is no debate over the fact that eating vegetables is healthy, but knowing that something is good for your health and knowing exactly how good it is for your health are two different things. Enter Victoria Kirsh, PhD. Dr. Kirsh is a graduate of the Yale School of Public Health and is currently a leading researcher on the relationship between diet and health. In 2007, Dr. Kirsh spearheaded a study to determine just how much of an impact eating fruits and vegetables can have in the prevention of prostate cancer.[1]

Looking at four years' worth of dietary and lifestyle data from 29,361 men in the Prostate, Lung, Colorectal, and Ovarian (PLCO) Cancer Screening Trial, Dr. Kirsh and her colleagues made some interesting discoveries. Overall vegetable consumption was found to have a significant inverse association with aggressive prostate cancer incidence. In other words, increasing vegetable, but not fruit, intake was significantly associated with a decrease in a study participant's risk for

40%

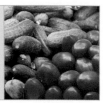

High vegetable intake reduced prostate cancer risk by up to 40% in a study evaluating the diets of nearly 30,000 men.

getting advanced prostate cancer.[1] Dr. Kirsh's findings showed that the study participants who consumed the most vegetables had a 40 percent reduction in their risk for aggressive prostate cancer incidence when compared to the participants consuming the fewest vegetables.

One unexpected, but important, finding from this study was that the biggest reduction in prostate cancer risk was primarily caused by one family of vegetables, the cruciferous vegetables.[1]

A similar study was led by Jennifer H. Cohen, PhD, MPH, a faculty member in the Department of Epidemiology at the University of Washington.[2] As we mentioned in chapter 1, epidemiology is the study of diseases, from how they originate to how they spread, and even how we can control them. For her Seattle-based study, Dr. Cohen and her team of researchers recruited 628 participants who had been newly diagnosed with prostate cancer and 602 age-matched healthy participants to compare their dietary practices and ultimately quantify the role of fruit and vegetable consumption in men's risk for getting prostate cancer. Supporting the results of Dr. Kirsh's study, Dr. Cohen's findings also indicated that while fruits did not have a significant impact in reducing the participants' risk for prostate cancer, vegetables did.[2] Again, like in Dr. Kirsh's study, Dr. Cohen and her team could not have foreseen the large role that cruciferous vegetables

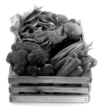

would play in their findings. In fact, cruciferous vegetables were found to account for the majority of the preventative nature of vegetable consumption. Dr. Cohen's study results showed that the men who had the highest overall vegetable intake reduced their risk by 35 percent. That said, the men

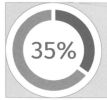

35%   41%

Study participants who ate the most vegetables decreased their risk for prostate cancer by 35%. This statistic jumped to 41% for participants who specifically had the highest intake of cruciferous vegetables.

who consumed three or more servings per week of specifically crucifer-ous vegetables bumped up that protective percentage to an impressive 41 percent reduction in prostate cancer risk![2]

Both of the studies we've discussed so far tell us nearly identical stories: men who consume diets rich in vegetables have significantly lower risk for prostate cancer. While it is not surprising that eating a lot of vegetables can decrease prostate cancer risk, the huge extent of risk reduction demonstrated by these two studies could not have been predicted. These studies showed that, by simply maintaining a diet high in veggies, men were able to cut their risk for aggressive prostate cancer nearly in half! The other unexpected aspect of these studies was the remarkable and unparalleled role that cruciferous vegetables played in reducing these men's risk for prostate cancer.

You may be currently asking yourself, "What are cruciferous vege-tables?" Cruciferous vegetables, or crucifers, are a nutrient-dense family of veggies that, according to the National Cancer Institute, include broccoli, cauliflower, brussels sprouts, cabbage, collard greens, kale, and turnips. In addition to the vegetables outlined by the National Cancer Institute, bok choy, daikon, and watercress are also part of this veggie subcategory.

While scientists began researching the connection between nutri-tion and prostate cancer by evaluating all fruits and vegetables, crucifers quickly made their way to the forefront of this area of research after several studies, including the two we have already discussed, found them to be a uniquely anti-cancer veggie family. The idea that a sin-gle group of vegetables could be a one-stop shop for reducing men's

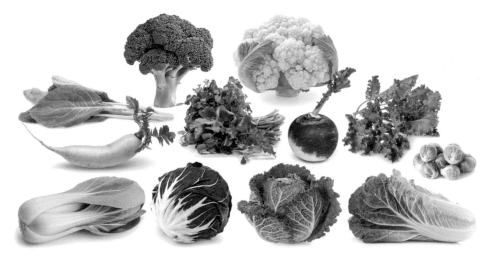

risk for prostate cancer was very appealing to the scientific community, which led to a new wave of research centered on crucifers. The goal of this new wave? Determine just how much power crucifers actually can have in prostate cancer prevention.

Researcher Astrid Steinbrecher, from the German Cancer Research Center, conducted one of these studies in the hopes of finding out the true impact of crucifers on men's risk for prostate cancer.[3] After following the dietary patterns of 11,405 study participants from the EPIC-Heidelberg cohort study for almost ten years, Steinbrecher's study found that as each participant's consumption of crucifers increased, their risk for prostate cancer decreased.[3] In fact, Steinbrecher and her team found that the men with the highest intake of crucifers alone (compared to the men with the lowest intake) were able to decrease their risk for prostate cancer by a statistically significant 32 percent.[3] The addition of this simple but powerful family of vegetables to these men's diets cut down their risk for prostate cancer by a third!

So, through a series of experiments and studies, researchers determined that crucifers have a superpower for preventing prostate cancer. But they didn't stop there. Next, researchers wanted to see if these vegetables could also destroy existing prostate cancer.

In a follow-up study, 1,560 men with nonmetastatic prostate cancer were recruited and their diets were tracked for six years.[4] The goal of this study was to determine how the progression of these men's cancer would be impacted by their consumption of cruciferous vegetables. Dietary data was collected from the participants every six months via food frequency questionnaires and medical reports. The study's findings were astounding. While the results showed that

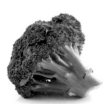

overall neither vegetable nor fruit consumptions were associated with reducing prostate cancer progression, the findings specifically related to cruciferous vegetable intake were quite different. Firstly, these researchers found that consuming cruciferous vegetables after prostate cancer

Can crucifers fight existing prostate cancer?

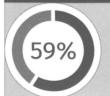

59%

Yes! While crucifers are heavy hitters in prostate cancer prevention, they are also powerful warriors in the fight against existing cancer. Studies show that high crucifer intake can decrease prostate cancer progression by up to 59%!

diagnosis was strongly associated with reduced risk of prostate cancer growth.[4] More exactly, these researchers found that the study participants who ate the most crucifers had 59 percent less cancer growth when compared to the men who had the lowest crucifer intake. Eating a handful of broccoli, kale, and brussels sprouts per day quite literally gave these men the ability to fight the progression of their cancer 59 percent more effectively than other men.[4]

At this point we have established that eating cruciferous vegetables can not only help prevent prostate cancer but also help people who already have prostate cancer reduce their cancer progression. Is there anything that crucifers cannot do? Let's just say for the sake of argument that these articles are cherry picked. After all, these findings do seem a little too good to be true, don't they? The interesting thing is, scientists were skeptical as well. It's hard to believe that a lifestyle change as simple as consuming more broccoli could reduce your risk for prostate cancer by over 30 percent. This disbelief led researchers to begin exploring the science behind why cruciferous vegetables have such powerful anti-cancer abilities.

Gregory Watson, PhD, pursued this exact topic when trying to ascertain which part of the cruciferous vegetable family was responsible for their anti-cancer properties.[5] In his meta-analysis, Dr. Watson collected the data from the best biochemical studies on the breakdown of crucifers at the molecular level. He found that crucifers contain compounds called glucosinolates, which are natural plant chemicals referred to in scientific literature as phytochemicals.[5] When consumed, the glucosinolates in cruciferous veggies break down in the body to smaller, active molecules that have strong cancer-fighting functions. These molecules are sulforaphane and indole-3-carbinol (I3C), and I3C also breaks down further into diindolylmethane (DIM). These three glucosinolate byproducts are the unique part of cruciferous vegetables that gives them their incredible anti-cancer properties. The mechanisms these molecules use to fight cancer in the human body include blocking the development of cancer cells by promoting detoxification, triggering cancer cell death through a process called apoptosis, and altering the genetic activity in cells that stop cancer from living and proliferating. Basically, the tiny molecules in crucifers have a big effect in (1) stopping cancer cells from multiplying and (2) killing off existing cancer cells.[5] These findings, compiled by Dr. Watson, are important because knowing the mechanisms cruciferous vegetables use to attack cancer helps explain why they are so good at preventing prostate cancer.

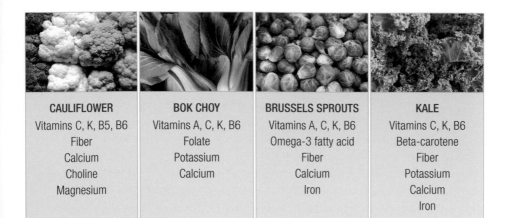

CAULIFLOWER	BOK CHOY	BRUSSELS SPROUTS	KALE
Vitamins C, K, B5, B6	Vitamins A, C, K, B6	Vitamins A, C, K, B6	Vitamins C, K, B6
Fiber	Folate	Omega-3 fatty acid	Beta-carotene
Calcium	Potassium	Fiber	Fiber
Choline	Calcium	Calcium	Potassium
Magnesium		Iron	Calcium
			Iron

In addition to glucosinolates, each vegetable in the cruciferous family also has a unique nutrient profile and therefore its own unique health benefits.

As if all the prostate cancer–related benefits are not enough, cruciferous vegetables have also been found to help prevent several other leading causes of death in the United States. As mentioned in chapter 1, heart disease is the number one killer of Americans, so let's start there. Xianglan Zhang, MD, MPH, from the Department of Medicine at Vanderbilt University Medical Center began researching the relationship between diet and heart disease in 2011.[6] Dr. Zhang could have looked at a handful of people to see how crucifer consumption would impact their risk for heart disease, or he could have looked at more than 100,000 people and explored the same topic. He chose the latter. Harnessing the dietary data of 134,796 participants in the Shanghai Men's Health Study and Shanghai Women's Health Study, Dr. Zhang aimed at determining the relationship between vegetables and mortality from cardiovascular disease. After a decade of follow-ups, Dr. Zhang and his colleagues found that the more veggies participants consumed, the better their cardiovascular health and the less likely they were to die from heart disease.[6] Specifically, the results indicated that as fruit and vegetable intake increased, the risk of death from both cardiovascular diseases and all-cause mortality decreased significantly. This outcome was true for all vegetables, but it was especially evident for cruciferous vegetable intake, which displayed a direct dose-response pattern with mortality. That means that the more cruciferous vegetables the participants ate, the greater their protection against dying from heart disease.

Continuing the long list of benefits associated with eating vegetables is another study that looked at the fifth leading cause of death in the United States, stroke.[7] Exploring the effects of fruit and vegetable intake on Americans' risk for ischemic stroke, this longitudinal study followed the diets of 114,279 Americans for more than ten years. Findings showed that the study participants who ate the most fruits and vegetables had a 31 percent lower risk for stroke, relative to those who consumed the least fruits and veggies.[7] Much like the findings from Dr. Zhang's study, these results were particularly pronounced when it specifically came to cruciferous vegetable intake. So essentially, eating vegetables, especially cruciferous ones, can decrease your risk for prostate cancer, heart disease, and stroke, to name just a few diseases.

Considering this information, you may now want to ask yourself, "Am I eating the ideal amount of veggies per day to reap all of these health benefits?"

If you are being honest with yourself, you probably aren't consuming enough vegetables. The Centers for Disease Control (CDC) has been kind enough to provide us with a reality based fact check when it comes to nutrition and the average American diet, in the form of a shocking statistic. In the most recent edition of the American Cancer Society's (ACS) guidelines for cancer prevention, they highlight the importance of vegetable consumption in reducing cancer risk.[8] The ACS guidelines for cancer prevention are a series of recommendations for leading a preventive lifestyle against cancer, formed using the current research available today on lifestyle practices and cancer. In their guidelines, the ACS discusses both the healthful practices you should be increasing and unhealthy practices you should decrease, including the best foods to eat and the optimal quantity of those foods to eat. In that vein, the ACS recommends that every adult consume two and a half cups of vegetables per day to achieve the ideal health benefits of this food group.

Based on this recommendation, the CDC conducted a nationwide compliance study to test if Americans were actually following this recommendation.[9] Their findings showed that less than 10 percent of Americans consume the recommended amount of two and a half cups of veggies every day. Less than 10 percent. Moreover, this statistic is a national average, so variation from state to state is significant.[9] For example, the CDC found that some states, such as West Virginia, have as few as 6 percent of adults who are meeting the ACS's vegetable consumption recommendation, while the District of Columbia, for instance, has 16 percent of adults meeting this recommendation.[9]

Finally, this study also found that vegetable intake levels are the lowest in young adults, adults facing poverty, and men.

The key to gaining the extensive healing effects that vegetables, like crucifers, can provide boils down to a single action: eating more vegetables! Specifically, eating the ACS's recommended two and a half cups of vegetables every day. There are additional, smaller actions you can take to ensure that you extract the most nutrition possible from the vegetables you consume, such as steaming your cruciferous veggies and chewing thoroughly before eating them.[10] It may seem odd that steamed veggies would be healthier than veggies in their raw form, but a study from 2018 found that when people ate steamed broccoli, they absorbed significantly more of the nutrients that make this vegetable so anti-cancerous: glucosinolates. In this study, people consumed broccoli that had been prepared in different ways to assess which preparation enabled the participants to absorb the most nutrients, and specifically the most glucosinolates. Study participants chewed either (1) steamed broccoli for eleven seconds, then thirty seconds, and finally forty seconds, or (2) both raw and steamed broccoli for twenty-two seconds. At the end of each prescribed time, the amount of glucosinolate absorbed by the participants was assessed. Findings showed that the highest glucosinolate concentrations resulted from the steamed samples that had been chewed for longer amounts of time.

But again, the most important step is getting those cancer-preventing veggies on your plate in the first place.

While this may not be an easy change to make, this action is straightforward. It is the choice to eat a hearty salad for lunch instead of a hamburger, or to pick a nutrient-dense, vegetable-based snack over calorie-dense chips. Individually, these actions are small and simple, but collectively they have the power to help you prevent prostate cancer and other diseases.

BIBLIOGRAPHY CHAPTER 2

1. Kirsh, V.A., Peters, U., Mayne, S.T., Subar, A.F., Chatterjee, N., Johnson, C.C, and Hayes, R.B. (2007). Prospective study of fruit and vegetable intake and risk of prostate cancer. *Journal of the National Cancer Institute,* 99(15):1200–1209. DOI:10.1093/jnci/djm065.

2. Cohen, J.H., Kristal, A.R., and Stanford, J.L. (2000). Fruit and vegetable intakes and prostate cancer risk. *Journal of the National Cancer Institute,* 92(1):61–68. DOI:10.1093/jnci/92.1.61.

3. Steinbrecher, A., Nimptsch, K., Hüsing, A., Rohrmann, S., and Linseisen, J. (2009). Dietary glucosinolate intake and risk of prostate cancer in the EPIC Heidelberg cohort study. *International Journal of Cancer,* 125(9):2179–2186. DOI:10.1002/ijc.24555.

4. Richman, E.L., Carroll, P.R., and Chan, J.M. (2012). Vegetable and fruit intake after diagnosis and risk of prostate cancer progression. *International Journal of Cancer,* 131(1):201–210. DOI:10.1002/ijc.26348.

5. Watson, G.W., Beaver, L.M., Williams, D.E., Dashwood, R.H., and Ho, E. (2013). Phytochemicals from cruciferous vegetables, epigenetics, and prostate cancer prevention. *The AAPS Journal,* 15(4):951–961. DOI:10.1208/s12248-013-9504-4.

6. Zhang, X., Shu, X.O., Xiang, Y.B., Yang, G., Li, H., Gao, J., and Zheng, W. (2011). Cruciferous vegetable consumption is associated with a reduced risk of total and cardiovascular disease mortality. *American Journal of Clinical Nutrition,* 94(1):240–246. DOI:10.3945/ajcn.110.009340.

7. Joshipura, K.J., Ascherio, A., Manson, J.E., Stampfer, M.J., Rimm, E.B., Speizer, F.E., Hennekens, C.H., et al. (1999). Fruit and vegetable intake in relation to risk of ischemic stroke. *JAMA,* 282(13):1233–1239. DOI:10.1001/jama.282.13.1233.

8. Kushi, L.H., Doyle, C., McCullough, M., Rock, C.L., Demark-Wahnefried, W., Bandera, E.V., Gapstur, S., et al. (2012). American Cancer Society guidelines on nutrition and physical activity for cancer prevention: reducing the risk of cancer with healthy food choices and physical activity. *CA: A Cancer Journal for Clinicians,* 62(1):30–67. DOI:10.3322/caac.20140.

9. "Only 1 in 10 Adults Get Enough Fruits or Vegetables." Centers for Disease Control and Prevention press release. November 16, 2017. www.cdc.gov/media/releases/2017/p1116-fruit-vegetable-consumption.html.

10. Sarvan, I., Van Der Klauw, M., Oliviero, T., Dekker, M., and Verkerk, R. (2018). The effect of chewing on oral glucoraphanin hydrolysis in raw and steamed broccoli. *Journal of Functional Foods,* 45:306–312. DOI:10.1016/j.jff.2018.04.033.

Additional Studies Not Detailed in the Chapter

11. Hardin, J., Cheng, I., and Witte, J.S. (2011). Impact of consumption of vegetable, fruit, grain, and high glycemic index foods on aggressive prostate cancer risk. *Nutrition and Cancer,* 63(6): 860–872. DOI:10.1080/01635581.2011.582224.
    To determine modifiable risk factors for aggressive prostate cancer, this study investigated the connection between diet and prostate cancer risk. Conducted in Cleveland, Ohio, this study looked at the diets of 982 men (470 of whom had been diagnosed with aggressive prostate cancer and 512 controls). When comparing participants with the highest intake of overall vegetables, and specifically leafy greens, to those with the lowest intake, findings showed that increasing both overall vegetable and leafy green intake were inversely associated with prostate cancer risk. More specifically, par-

ticipants with the highest intake of both had a 34 percent decreased risk for aggressive prostate cancer in comparison to participants with the lowest intake. Findings from this study suggest that diets high in vegetables can potentially lower men's risk for the development of aggressive prostate cancer.

12. Kolonel, L.N., Hankin, J.H., Whittemore, A.S., Wu, A.H., Gallagher, R.P., Wilkens, L.R., John, E.M., et al. (2000). Vegetables, fruits, legumes, and prostate cancer: a multiethnic case-control study. *Cancer Epidemiology Biomarkers and Prevention*, 9(8):795–804. https://cebp.aacrjournals.org/content/9/8/795.full-text.pdf.

As a multiethnic study, this experiment not only explored the association between diet and prostate cancer risk but also considered an additional variable: ethnicity. Data for this study was collected via population-based registries, with 1,619 subjects being matched by age, region, and ethnicity to 1,618 controls. After analysis, the results showed a 39 percent decrease in prostate cancer risk for subjects with the highest consumption of cruciferous vegetables when compared to subjects with the lowest consumption. Interestingly enough, these findings were consistent across ethnic groups, suggesting the generally protective effects of crucifers against prostate cancer incidence.

13. Traka, M., Gasper, A.V., Melchini, A., Bacon, J.R., Needs, P.W., Frost, V., Chantry, A., et al. (2008). Broccoli consumption interacts with GSTM1 to perturb oncogenic signaling pathways in the prostate. *PLOS One*, 3(7):e2568. DOI:10.1371/journal.pone.0002568.

Looking at alterations in gene expression in men's prostate glands after a broccoli-rich diet, this study uniquely explores the impact of cruciferous vegetables on prostate cancer risk at the molecular level. Twenty-two subjects with high-grade prostatic intraepithelial neoplasia were given a broccoli-rich diet to consume for one year. Gene expression was evaluated at six months, as well as one year into the dietary intervention, with subjects' baseline gene expression acting as controls. Alterations in gene expression observed after intervention included changes to mRNA processing, TGFB1, EGF, and insulin signaling. The complex changes observed in prostate gland gene expression are associated with signaling pathways involved in prostate inflammation and carcinogenesis. This study is the first of its kind to provide gene-based evidence that cruciferous vegetables may reduce men's risk for prostate cancer.

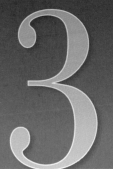

Tomatoes and Lycopene

S lice 'em, dice 'em, turn 'em into paste. Raw or cooked. Canned or fresh. There is no wrong way to eat the tomato, a nutrient-packed superfood, and the star of this chapter. Before we dive in, let's see how well you know your tomatoes.

CHERRY TOMATOES
These crisp, bite-sized tomatoes are perfect for snacking and adding to salads.

ROMA TOMATOES
The tanginess of these juicy tomatoes makes them great for canning and sauces.

TOMATOES ON THE VINE
Still attached to the vine they grew on, these hearty tomatoes are just as delicious raw as they are canned.

BEEFSTEAK TOMATOES
The mild flavor of these large, meaty tomatoes complements any sandwich.

HEIRLOOM TOMATOES
Coming in a variety of bright colors and sizes, these tomatoes range in flavor from sweet to earthy.

According to the United States Department of Agriculture Food Availability and Consumption data report, tomatoes are the second most commonly consumed vegetable in the United States, second only to potatoes. Interestingly enough, this is mainly due to Americans' high intake of pizza sauce, which accounted for 56 percent of the tomatoes consumed by Americans.[1] While pizza is probably not the best way to get your daily dose of tomatoes, it is important for you to find a way to fit tomatoes into your diet, and here's why: as a superfood, tomatoes are packed with micronutrients and natural plant chemicals known as phytochemicals.[2] From a nutrition perspective, tomatoes are an excellent source of potassium, folate, and vitamins A, C, and E. From the phytochemical perspective, tomatoes contain polyphenols and carotenoids, including beta-carotene and lycopene, the compound that gives tomatoes their bright red color. Lycopene also happens to be a very powerful antioxidant.[2] Because of the tomato's unique nutritional profile, research has indicated that consuming this superfood may help reduce your risk for prostate cancer.[2-6] As usual, we won't make you take our word on the matter, especially not when there is a wealth of studies to explore on this topic.

Edward Giovannucci, MD, ScD, a scientific leader in the world of nutrition and cancer, initiated one such study. Currently, Dr. Giovannucci is a professor of nutrition and epidemiology at the Harvard T.H. Chan School of Public Health. He is also the editor in chief of the recognized and respected journal *Cancer Causes and Control*, and an avid researcher on the various factors that contribute to cancer incidence. In 2002, Dr. Giovannucci decided to investigate the connection between tomato consumption and men's risk for prostate cancer.[3] In his pursuit of this subject, Dr. Giovannucci decided to conduct a prospective study using dietary and lifestyle data reported by more than 47,000 participants in the Health Professionals Follow-Up Study. Data from these participants was collected via food frequency questionnaires over a twelve-year period, after which point it was analyzed by Dr. Giovannucci and his team of researchers. After analysis, the results of his study showed a significant inverse association between tomato intake and prostate cancer risk. This

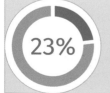

23%

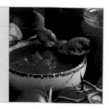

Study participants who enjoyed two or more servings of tomato sauce per week had a 23% lower risk for prostate cancer incidence.

association was even stronger for aggressive forms of prostate cancer. This means that as the participants in this study increased the amount of tomatoes they ate, their risk for getting prostate cancer decreased. Specifically, the men in this study who consumed two or more servings of tomato sauce per week were found to have a 23 percent reduced risk for prostate cancer and a 35 percent decreased risk for aggressive prostate cancer, in comparison to those who consumed fewer than one serving of tomatoes a month.[3] These findings demonstrate that an increase in tomato intake can, in fact, reduce men's risk for prostate cancer.[3]

For this study, Dr. Giovannucci chose to look at tomato sauce in particular because other research has indicated that the way tomatoes are processed may change the types and amounts of micronutrients and phytochemicals available when this fruit is consumed. For example, when tomatoes are in a canned or sauce form, they provide the best source of the antioxidant lycopene.

In 2002, during the time of Dr. Giovannucci's study, lycopene was just beginning to be explored for its unique anti-cancer properties. Therefore, although this study was centered on tomato consumption in general, it also kick-started a fascination within the cancer research community on the specific impact of lycopene.

If you are like me, you are now thinking, "That's great, but Dr. Giovannucci's findings are so 2002," and you are right—in some cases, newer data can be better data. So let's take a look at a second study that was conducted more than a decade after Dr. Giovannucci's study. Following in the footsteps of Dr. Giovannucci, epidemiologist Kirsten Zu, PhD, a graduate of the Harvard T.H. Chan School of Public Health, led a second study. An accomplished researcher, Dr. Zu specializes in nutrition, cancer pathology, and riskassessment studies. Several years ago, Dr. Zu became interested in the impact of nutrition on men's risk for prostate cancer.

Dr. Zu wanted to understand if there was a connection between eating tomatoes and prostate cancer risk in men. Dr. Zu and her colleagues decided to take Dr. Giovannucci's work to the next level by focusing on the unique role that

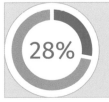
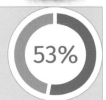

Higher lycopene intake is associated with a significant reduction in risk: a 28% reduction in risk for prostate cancer incidence and a 53% reduction in risk for lethal prostate cancer incidence.

28%

53%

the lycopene in tomatoes might play in men's risk for getting prostate cancer.[4] Dr. Zu used a subset of data from the Health Professionals Follow-Up Study for her study. Specifically, Dr. Zu's research included dietary information from nearly fifty thousand participants whose lifestyles were followed for a four-year period. What Dr. Zu and her team found was striking. Results showed that the higher participants' lycopene intake was, the lower their risk for getting prostate cancer became. In fact, the study participants with the highest lycopene intake reduced their risk for prostate cancer by 28 percent, when compared to participants with the lowest lycopene intake![4] What's more, these findings were even stronger when it came to reducing men's risk for lethal prostate cancer incidence.[4] In other words, lycopene not only decreased participants' likelihood of getting prostate cancer but also even more strongly decreased their likelihood of dying from prostate cancer. The findings from this study reinforced those of Dr. Giovannucci by providing further support for the theory that tomatoes, and the lycopene found in tomatoes, have the potential to significantly decrease your risk for prostate cancer.

We have established that tomatoes have the power to reduce your risk of prostate cancer incidence; now it's time to understand where this power comes from. As we mentioned at the beginning of this chapter, tomatoes contain phytochemicals, like lycopene, which makes them strong antioxidants. But what is an antioxidant and why are antioxidants important players in cancer prevention?

Think of the trillions of cells in your body as tiny machines in an assembly line. When all of the machines are working normally, the assembly line can successfully create products. Unfortunately, like any machine, our cells do not always function perfectly. Sometimes, a cell will carry out a process flawlessly 1,000 times, but on the 1,001st time, something goes wrong. One of the ways that things go wrong in our cells is when they create reactive oxygen species (ROS).[5] ROS are the defective products of normal cellular processes gone wrong, harmful lifestyle activities, and unhealthy dietary choices. ROS react with normal things in our cells, like our DNA, and cause oxidative damage. Oxidative damage has been implicated in the origins of many chronic diseases, including prostate cancer.[5] If ROS are the supervillains in the fight between healthy cells and cancerous cells, antioxidants are the superheroes. Antioxidants are protective molecules that destroy ROS. They do this by reducing reactive oxygen species, decreasing oxidative damage, and increasing antioxidant potential. In these ways, antioxidants can delay and even prevent oxidative damage caused by ROS that leads to cancer and other diseases.[5]

In addition to their antioxidant properties, tomatoes also use a few other biochemical mechanisms to prevent prostate cancer. In a recently published literature review, Kirstie Canene-Adams, PhD, and her colleagues at the Department of Food Science and Human Nutrition at the University of Illinois determined several biological pathways that compounds in tomatoes use to help your body destroy cancer cells. These pathways include the exertion of anti-growth factor effects and the inhibition of cancer cell proliferation (reproduction and growth). A meta-analysis published by the *Canadian Medical Association Journal* expanded on Dr. Canene-Adam's review by delving into the more technical mechanisms tomato compounds use to protect our bodies from cancer, including immune modulation, gene function regulation, and gap-junction communication. That said, antioxidants are still considered tomatoes' star fighters in the battle royal against prostate cancer.

So how can you stock up on as many antioxidants as possible? Easy: antioxidants abound in many fruits and vegetables! Some of the antioxidants you consume when you eat a tomato are vitamins E and C, various polyphenols, and lycopene.[2] Lycopene is by far the strongest antioxidant on this list. Plants naturally produce lycopene, but unfortunately the human body cannot.[2] Therefore, to get the great health benefits associated with lycopene, you must include it in your diet. The best way to do this is by eating tomatoes. In fact, 80 percent of the lycopene in Americans' diets comes from tomatoes. While tomatoes are the best source of dietary lycopene, other sources are watermelons, pink grapefruits, and pink guava.

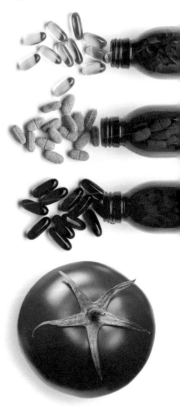

Now you may be thinking, "If lycopene is the best part of the tomato, why don't I just cut straight to the chase and take a lycopene supplement, instead of eating tomatoes whole?" Although lycopene is a key player in tomatoes' ability to fight prostate cancer, it isn't the only player. Studies have shown that consuming tomatoes whole is better at destroying cancer than is consuming lycopene extract alone.[2] Scientists think this is because of the many other important antioxidants, phytochemicals, and micronutrients that can be found in whole tomatoes that aren't present in a lycopene extract. You could take a supplemental pill for lycopene, another one for vitamin E, and a third one for vitamin C, and those three pills still won't have the same holistic impact on your health as eating one tomato in its entirety.

That said, there are a few things you can do when eating tomatoes to maximize the lycopene your body obtains from this superfood. For starters, you can learn from Dr. Giovannucci's study, which taught us that tomato sauce is the most bioavailable source of lycopene.[2] "Bio-availability" is a term used to describe the amount of nutrients that is actually absorbed and used by your body when you consume a given food. Therefore, when we say tomato sauce is the most bioavailable source of lycopene, what we mean is that when you eat tomatoes in sauce form, your body is able to absorb more nutrients, like lycopene, than it would if the tomato was in another form. In addition to eating tomatoes in sauce form, you can also increase the amount of lycopene your body absorbs from this superfood if you combine it with olive oil.[6]

The benefits of combining olive oil and tomatoes was, in part, discovered by a study conducted in the early 2000s, which found that dicing and cooking tomatoes with olive oil could significantly increase the bioavailability of lycopene. Twenty-three individuals were recruited for this study. For nearly two weeks, half of the participants ate tomatoes that had been diced and then cooked in olive oil, while the other half ate diced, cooked tomatoes without olive oil. At the end of the study, blood samples were drawn from all participants to see which group had the highest concentration of lycopene in their system. After analysis, the participants who had olive oil added to their tomatoes had up to 82 percent more lycopene in their blood when compared to those who ate the tomatoes without olive oil. Based on their findings, these researchers concluded that adding extra-virgin olive oil to diced tomatoes while cooking significantly increases lycopene absorption. This conclusion also reinforces that the way tomatoes are prepared and processed helps determine the bioavailability of this superfood's micronutrients and phytochemicals.

A physician-approved nutritional recipe that includes this combo is the simple and delicious Four-Ingredient Mediterranean Salad on page 31.

In the previous chapter we explored the impact of vegetables and crucifers on your risk for prostate cancer. In this chapter we discussed the same topic, but with tomatoes. There is compelling data that each of these foods alone can help you prevent prostate cancer, but what would happen if we combined them? What if instead of looking at the impact of broccoli *or* tomatoes on reducing your risk for cancer, we looked at the impact of broccoli *and* tomatoes together?

In a preliminary study on this topic, animal models with prostate cancer were fed one of the following meal plans for a twenty-two-week

Four-Ingredient Mediterranean Salad

4 Roma tomatoes, diced

1 large English or Persian cucumber, diced

¼ red onion, diced

1½ tablespoons extra-virgin olive oil

Freshly squeezed juice from ½ lemon
(about 2 tablespoons)

Salt

Ground black pepper

Put the tomatoes, cucumber, and onion in a large
salad bowl. Add the oil and lemon juice and toss until
evenly distributed. Season with salt and pepper to taste,
toss again gently, and serve.

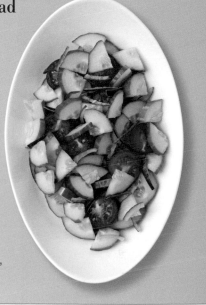

period: (1) added tomatoes, (2) added broccoli, (3) added tomatoes and broccoli, or (4) added lycopene extract.[7] After the twenty-two weeks were up, the tumors were removed from their animal models and analyzed. Findings showed that while the first diet had reduced the animals' prostate tumor growth by 34 percent and the second diet had reduced the prostate tumor growth by 42 percent, the third diet boosted this percentage to an astounding 52 percent reduction in tumor growth.[7] By simply adding tomatoes and broccoli to their diets, the participants in this study were able to cut their tumor growth in half! There is no question that tomatoes alone made an impact in reducing tumor growth, as did broccoli alone. But you cannot beat the combined effect of adding *both* tomatoes and broccoli to your diet when it comes to reducing prostate cancer growth and development.

In addition to the anti-cancer properties of tomatoes, increasing your consumption of this superfood can also help you prevent other major diseases. Why don't we start by looking at the impact of tomatoes on your risk for heart disease, the leading cause of death in the United States? In a multicenter, case-controlled study conducted across ten European countries, researchers found that tomatoes, and lycopene specifically, were directly tied to lowering people's risk for myocardial infarctions, or heart attacks.[8] After analysis, the results revealed that

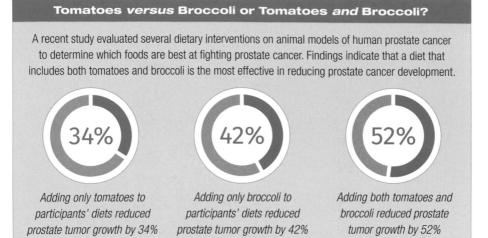

Tomatoes *versus* Broccoli or Tomatoes *and* Broccoli?

A recent study evaluated several dietary interventions on animal models of human prostate cancer to determine which foods are best at fighting prostate cancer. Findings indicate that a diet that includes both tomatoes and broccoli is the most effective in reducing prostate cancer development.

34%

Adding only tomatoes to participants' diets reduced prostate tumor growth by 34%

42%

Adding only broccoli to participants' diets reduced prostate tumor growth by 42%

52%

Adding both tomatoes and broccoli reduced prostate tumor growth by 52%

lycopene was actually the only carotenoid (plant pigment) to be significantly associated with reducing a participant's risk for heart attacks. Not only were tomatoes associated with a reduced risk, but findings from this study revealed that the participants with the highest intake of tomatoes were able to cut their risk for getting a heart attack quite literally in half when compared to those with the lowest tomato intake.[8] These participants literally reduced their risk for a heart attack by 50 percent, just by choosing to eat more tomatoes every day.

Surprisingly, the magnitude of this finding is mirrored in studies that look at dietary intake of tomatoes and stroke risk as well. A decade-long study in Finland looked at the dietary patterns of 1,031 to determine the true association between eating tomatoes and stroke risk. While many studies get dietary data from their participants via food frequency questionnaires, this study took a unique, more exact approach by measuring their participants' tomato consumption via the amount of lycopene in their blood.[9] Their findings were remarkable. Results showed that participants with the lowest tomato intake had more than double the risk for having a stroke when compared to those who ate the most tomatoes.[9] Based on the findings from these studies, not only can tomatoes significantly reduce your risk for prostate cancer, but high tomato intake may also halve your risk for both heart attacks and strokes.

Combine the findings from all of these studies and one thing is clear. Tomatoes have the potential to significantly reduce your risk for many chronic and life-threatening diseases: prostate cancer, heart disease, and stroke included. Although studies on this topic generally support this

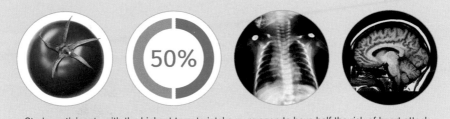

Study participants with the highest tomato intake were seen to have half the risk of heart attack or stroke when compared to those with the lowest intake of tomatoes.

statement, not all studies on tomatoes and prostate cancer are unanimous in their findings. You should note that some studies have not found an association between tomatoes and prostate cancer risk.[10–12]

Two such studies, both conducted in 2000, aimed at determining the impact that fruit and vegetable intake would have on men's prostate cancer risk.[10, 11] After evaluating dietary data from their relatively small number of participants, the scientists in these studies were not able to find significant connections between tomato intake and prostate cancer incidence. On the other hand, both studies found that the participants who ate the most vegetables had significantly decreased risk for prostate cancer incidence.[10, 11]

A third study from 2006 evaluated the diets from a much larger sample size but also did not find a significant connection between tomatoes and prostate cancer risk.[12] Looking at lifestyle and dietary data from 29,361 men for an average of 4.2 years, this study aimed at understanding the association between tomatoes, lycopene, and prostate cancer risk. With 1,338 cases of prostate cancer diagnosed over the study's follow-up period, these men had an incidence rate of 4.6 percent (less than half the national incidence rate).[12] The results showed that lycopene, tomatoes, and tomato-based products did not reduce the participants' risk for getting prostate cancer. This observed insignificant connection between tomatoes and prostate cancer risk could, in part, be due to the participants' atypically low incidence rate of prostate cancer, which could make associations more difficult to demonstrate.[12]

While it is important to recognize these outlier studies, it is perhaps more important to recognize that our research has not identified a single article that displays any detrimental effects from eating tomatoes. At best, current research indicates that eating more tomatoes can significantly reduce your risk for prostate cancer, and at worst you are just eating more of a delicious and nutritious food.

BIBLIOGRAPHY CHAPTER 3

1. "Food Availability and Consumption." U.S. Department of Agriculture, Economic Research Service. Accessed November 14, 2019. www.ers.usda.gov/data-products/ag-and-food-statistics-charting-the-essentials/food-availability-and-consumption.

2. Canene-Adams, K., Campbell, J.K., Zaripheh, S., Jeffery, E.H., and Erdman, J.W. (2005). The tomato as a functional food. *The Journal of Nutrition*, 135(5): 1226–1230. DOI:10.1093/jn/135.5.1226.

3. Giovannucci, E., Rimm, E.B., Liu, Y., Stampfer, M.J., and Willett, W.C. (2002). A prospective study of tomato products, lycopene, and prostate cancer risk. *Journal of the National Cancer Institute*, 94(5):391–398. DOI:10.1093/jnci/94.5.391.

4. Zu, K., Mucci, L., Rosner, B.A., Clinton, S.K., Loda, M., Stampfer, M.J., and Giovannucci, E. (2014). Dietary lycopene, angiogenesis, and prostate cancer: A prospective study in the prostate-specific antigen era. *Journal of the National Cancer Institute*, 106(2):djt430. DOI:10.1093/jnci/djt430.

5. Agarwal, S. and Rao, A.V. (2000). Tomato lycopene and its role in human health and chronic diseases. *Canadian Medical Association Journal*, 163(6):739–744. PMID:11022591.

6. Fielding J.M., Rowley, K.G., Cooper, P., and O'Dea, K. (2005). Increases in plasma lycopene concentration after consumption of tomatoes cooked with olive oil. *Asia Pacific Journal of Clinical Nutrition*, 14(2):131–136. PMID:15927929.

7. Canene-Adams, K., Lindshield, B.L., Wang, S., Jeffery, E.H., Clinton, S.K., and Erdman, J.W. (2007). Combinations of tomato and broccoli enhance antitumor activity in dunning R3327-H prostate adenocarcinomas. *Cancer Research*, 67(2): 836-842. DOI:10.1158/0008-5472.CAN-06-3462.

8. Kohlmeier, L., Kark, J.D., Gomez-Gracia, E., Martin, B.C., Steck, S.E., Kardinaal, A.F., Ringstad, J., et al. (1997). Lycopene and myocardial infarction risk in the EURAMIC Study. *American Journal of Epidemiology*, 146(8):618–626. DOI:10.1093/oxfordjournals.aje.a009327.

9. Karppi, J., Laukkanen, J.A., Sivenius, J., Ronkainen, K., and Kurl, S. (2012). Serum lycopene decreases the risk of stroke in men: A population-based follow-up study. *Neurology*, 79(15):1540–1547. DOI:10.1212/WNL.0b013e31826e26a6.

10. Cohen, J.H., Kristal, A.R., and Stanford, J.L. (2000). Fruits and vegetable intakes and prostate cancer risk. *Journal of the National Cancer Institute*, 92(1):61–68. DOI:10.1093/jnci/92.1.61.

11. Kolonel, L.N., Hankin, J.H., Whittemore, A.S., Wu, A.H., Gallagher, R.P, Wilkens, L.R., John, E.M., et al. (2000). Vegetables, fruits, legumes, and prostate cancer: a multiethnic case-control study. *Cancer Epidemiology, Biomarkers and Prevention*, 9(8):795–804.

12. Kirsh, V.A., Mayne, S.T., Peters, U., Chatterjee, N., Leitzmann, M.F., Dixon, L.B, Urban, D.A., et al. (2006). A prospective study of lycopene and tomato product intake and risk of prostate cancer. *Cancer Epidemiology, Biomarkers and Prevention*, 15(1):92–98. DOI:10.1158/1055-9965.EPI-05-0563.

Soy

Soybeans are one of the most important legumes in the world.[1] Native to East Asia, this nutrient-dense bean has provided people with a vegetable-based protein source for thousands of years. While soybeans were a staple in East Asian cuisine far before written records existed, some of our earliest records of soybeans date back to 7000 BCE China, where the soybean was considered a sacred plant.[1] It wasn't until the eighteenth century that soybeans found their way to the United States, by way of Samuel Bowen and James Flint, the first Englishmen legally allowed to learn Chinese.[2] At first, these precious legumes were solely used by Americans to produce farm animal feed, but, after scientists realized the immense nutritional value of these legumes in the early 1900s, soybeans became one of America's largest, most versatile farm crops. Today, soybeans are the second-largest cash crop in the United States.[2]

Soybeans are consumed in many forms, ranging from whole to fermented. Common soybean products include edamame (green soybeans), soy milk, tofu (bean curd), soy sauce, miso (soybean paste), natto (fermented soybeans), tempeh, soy flour, and soybean oil.[1] Below is a flow chart detailing the various processes the raw bean undergoes to produce the commercial soybean products we regularly consume.

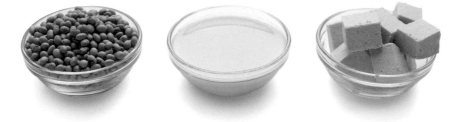

Processing Soybeans from Raw to Finished Products

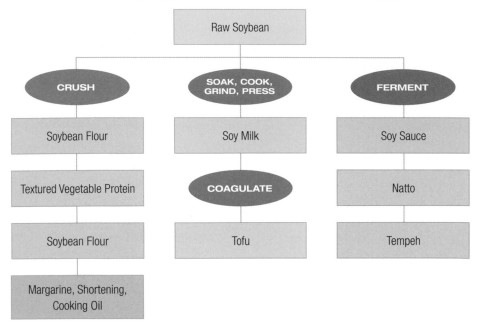

While the soybean is now consumed globally, as we mentioned earlier, it originated in East Asia where to this day it is still a major ingredient in daily meals. The high intake of soybeans and soy products in Asian countries is unsurprising because this small legume packs a big nutritional punch. In addition to being an excellent source of protein, soy is rich in fiber, folate, calcium, iron, and potassium.[1] Soybeans also contain important organic molecules called isoflavones. So, what are isoflavones?

Isoflavones are a type of polyphenolic compound. Polyphenols are secondary metabolites only produced by plants, meaning your body cannot produce them. Studies have found that polyphenols, and isoflavones specifically, are beneficial for human health. These compounds have been implicated in the prevention of many diseases, including heart disease, type 2 diabetes, and prostate cancer.[4]

Because the human body cannot make isoflavones on its own, the only way for us to obtain these molecules is through our diet. Luckily, soybeans are the single best way to incorporate isoflavones into your daily diet.[4] Soybeans contain an abundance of isoflavones, with every 100 grams of soybeans containing anywhere from 5 to 30 milligrams of this powerful polyphenol. Isoflavones are so good for us because they have serious anti-cancer properties.[4-6] Isoflavones use three main mechanisms to protect our bodies from cancer. The first mechanism is the "hormone-like" effects isoflavones have on prostate cancer cells, which result in the isoflavones blocking the cancer cell from growing.[4] The second mechanism is the "nonhormone-like" effects isoflavones have on cancer cells, which basically halt cancer replication and initiate cancer cell death. Finally, isoflavones are strong antioxidants, and as we know from earlier chapters, antioxidants are cancer-fighting warriors.[5]

Several studies have been conducted to show the range and impressive capacity isoflavones have for destroying prostate cancer cells. One of these studies was led by the researcher Renea Taylor (née Jarred), PhD, a researcher at the Monash Biomedicine Discovery Institute. Dr. Taylor's research specialty is prostate cancer, and she is actually the chair of an initiative that supports research to improve treatments and clinical management for men with prostate cancer. In the early 2000s, Dr. Taylor chose to conduct a study on whether or not isoflavones would have an effect on prostate cancer.[6] Specifically, Dr. Taylor wanted to explore if isoflavones could help induce cancer cell death in men with prostate cancer.

For her study, Dr. Taylor recruited thirty-eight men with low- to moderate-grade prostate cancer and split them into two groups: a treatment group and a control group. The men in the treatment group took a 160-milligram isoflavone supplement every day for up to seven weeks, while the control group received a placebo pill. After the seven weeks were up, prostate samples were taken from all participants. These prostate specimens were then analyzed and the relative numbers of prostate cancer cells that had been destroyed throughout the study was recorded. The goal was to see if the soy treatment would help improve men's ability to kill prostate cancer cells. The findings were extraordinary.

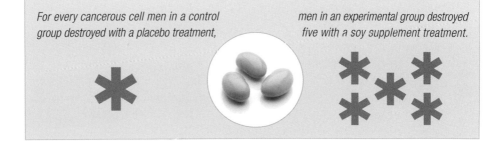

For every cancerous cell men in a control group destroyed with a placebo treatment, men in an experimental group destroyed five with a soy supplement treatment.

While the men from the control group destroyed an average of 0.25 percent of their cancer cells, the men from the treatment group had killed an average of 1.48 percent of their cancer cells.[6] That means that the men who took the isoflavone treatment eliminated five times more prostate cancer cells when compared to the men who did not have the isoflavone treatment! An additional, unexpected finding was that while the rates of cancer cell death in treated men was significantly higher than that of untreated men, this result was especially pronounced in the men with low to moderate stages of cancer. This study is a prime example of the power of isoflavones in action. These findings suggest that adding foods high in isoflavones, like soybeans, to your diet may help slow down low- to moderate-stage prostate cancer development and progression by way of cancer cell death.[6]

We know that soybeans contain potent anti-cancer properties and we also know that they are a dietary staple in many Asian countries. Putting two and two together led scientists to a new hypothesis: perhaps Asian countries have such a low rate of prostate cancer incidence because their populations eat a lot of soy. This hypothesis was the driving force behind many studies that have been conducted across Asia over the years to evaluate the relationship between soy intake and prostate cancer risk.

The largest study on this topic was organized by Norie Kurahashi, MD, from the National Cancer Center in Japan. An avid contributor to the world of prostate cancer research, Dr. Kurahashi has published countless studies on the relationship between diet and prostate cancer. As such, leading a study on the impact of soy intake on prostate cancer risk was well within Dr. Kurahashi's wheelhouse of expertise.[7] For this study, Dr. Kurahashi and her colleagues evaluated nine years' worth of data on the diets of more than forty thousand Japanese men in the Japan Public Health Center-based Prospective Study (JPHC Study). During the study's follow-up period, 307 cases of prostate cancer were recorded. Before analyzing the data, Dr. Kurahashi and her team chose to limit the data to only men over the age of sixty. Dr. Kurahashi made some fascinating observations.

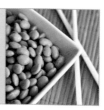

48% Participants with the highest soy intake decreased their risk for localized prostate cancer incidence by a whopping 48%.

Results showed that eating soy was significantly linked with a reduced risk for prostate cancer in study participants over the age of sixty.[7] In fact, soy foods and isoflavone intake were both associated with a dose-dependent decrease in localized prostate cancer risk. Put simply, the more soy products and isoflavones men ate, the proportionally lower their risk for localized prostate cancer became. The participants who consumed the most soy were able to decrease their risk for localized prostate cancer by a whopping 48 percent when compared to men eating the least soy.[7] When Dr. Kurahashi looked at the intake of soy isoflavones specifically, the protective effects against prostate cancer that had been observed with soy foods was mirrored. This finding indicates that isoflavones may be the unique part of soy that gives this superfood its anti-cancer properties. Based on these extraordinary findings, it appears that eating more soy foods can possibly cut your risk for localized prostate cancer nearly in half!

Oddly enough, while eating soy and soy products reduced the study participants' risk for localized prostate cancer incidence, it did not significantly reduce their risk for advanced prostate cancer.[7] In other words, eating soy protected men from the early stages of prostate cancer but was useless against the more advanced stages of this disease. How is it possible that soy, and specifically the isoflavones in soy, can have such a positive impact on fighting early-stage prostate cancer, but not the later stages?

To explain this odd observation, we need to dive a little deeper into how soy protects the body from prostate cancer. As we discussed earlier, the main way isoflavones fight prostate cancer is through "hormone-like" effects. These hormone-like effects are a result of the fact that isoflavones are a plant-derived version of estrogen.[4] Estrogen is a hormone that normally functioning human bodies produce regularly. To process and use the estrogen we produce, there are specific locations on cells throughout our bodies where the estrogen can bind. As plant versions of estrogen, isoflavones also have the ability to bind to the estrogen-specific binding sites within our body, which include those on prostate cells in prostate tissue. When isoflavones bind to these estrogen-specific sites, they are able to fight against the development of prostate cancer.

In the early stages of prostate cancer, prostate tissue has estrogen-specific binding sites, just like healthy prostate tissue does, so the isoflavones in soy can effectively help fight against the cancer.[7] But, as prostate cancer progresses to more advanced stages, studies have found

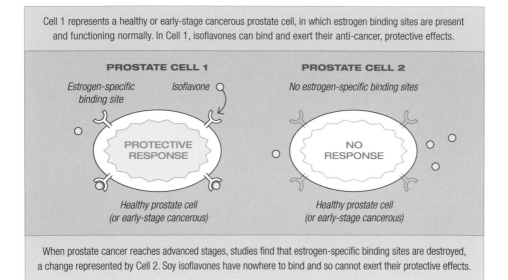

Cell 1 represents a healthy or early-stage cancerous prostate cell, in which estrogen binding sites are present and functioning normally. In Cell 1, isoflavones can bind and exert their anti-cancer, protective effects.

PROSTATE CELL 1

Estrogen-specific binding site   Isoflavone

PROTECTIVE RESPONSE

Healthy prostate cell (or early-stage cancerous)

PROSTATE CELL 2

No estrogen-specific binding sites

NO RESPONSE

Healthy prostate cell (or early-stage cancerous)

When prostate cancer reaches advanced stages, studies find that estrogen-specific binding sites are destroyed, a change represented by Cell 2. Soy isoflavones have nowhere to bind and so cannot exert their protective effects.

that prostate tissue will partially or completely lose its estrogen-specific binding sites. If the prostate tissue loses its estrogen binding sites, then the soy isoflavones cannot bind, and therefore they cannot protect the tissue from cancer.[7] This biological process could explain why studies have found that soy has the ability to reduce men's risk only for early-stage, localized prostate cancer incidence.

Other studies on the subject of soy and prostate cancer have been conducted on a smaller scale than Dr. Kurahashi's study, but they have by and large come to similar conclusions. Eating more soy could decrease men's risk for getting prostate cancer.

In China, a study compared the diets of men with prostate cancer to the diets of healthy men to see if soy (and isoflavone) intake played a role in prostate cancer risk.[8] To accomplish this goal, these Chinese scientists recruited 133 men with prostate cancer and 265 healthy men and then collected data about their diets via interviews and food frequency questionnaires over a three-year period. After analyzing the

49% Studies have found that eating soy may decrease your risk for prostate cancer by up to 49%.

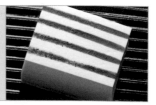

diets of the nearly four hundred study participants, these researchers found that soy consumption, and the intake of isoflavones in particular, significantly decreased men's risk for prostate cancer. Men with the highest soy food intake had a 49 percent smaller chance of getting prostate cancer than participants with the lowest intake.[8]

Furthermore, the men consuming the highest quantity of isoflavones also had up to a 47 percent reduction in prostate cancer risk. A Japanese study used a similar format to compare the diets of 140 men with prostate cancer to 140 healthy men to determine the impact of soy intake on men's risk for this disease.[8] The results showed that the consumption of soybean products was significantly associated with a decreased risk for prostate cancer. Participants who ate the most soybean products had a 47 percent lower risk for prostate cancer than those who ate the least soybean products.[9] This significant risk reduction was reflected when researchers looked specifically at tofu (bean curd) and natto (fermented soybean) consumption. In fact, men eating the most tofu had a 53 percent reduction in risk and men eating the most natto had a 75 percent risk reduction when compared to those eating the least tofu and natto, respectively.[9] The findings from both these studies further reinforce Dr. Kurahashi's conclusion that soy foods and isoflavones may play a role in reducing men's risk for prostate cancer.

While countless studies have found that soybeans, soy products, and isoflavones may significantly decrease men's risk for prostate cancer, it is also important to recognize the handful of valid studies that have found no connection between soy intake and prostate cancer incidence.

A prime example of a valid study that did not find a connection between eating soy and prostate cancer was led by Song-Yi Park, PhD, a researcher at the University of Hawaii Cancer Center.[10] For this study, Dr. Park analyzed the dietary data from men in the Multiethnic Cohort Study (MEC) to determine the relationship between legumes, soy, and isoflavone intake and prostate cancer risk in men. The MEC is a large-scale, longitudinal prospective study of Hawaiian and Californian residents aimed at better understanding the factors that contribute to the development of cancer and other chronic diseases. Of the 215,000 participants in the MEC, 82,483 fit the criteria for the study at hand. Dietary data from these participants was collected via food frequency questionnaires over an average follow-up of eight years. Over the course of this eight-year period, 4,404 cases of prostate cancer were recorded. Findings from this study showed that while the participants who ate the most soy decreased their risk for prostate cancer by 10 percent, this percentage was statistically insignificant.[10] When a statistic is insignificant it means there is a possibility that the observed association was due to chance and not actually the result of a real connection.

A possible explanation for this insignificant finding is that the food frequency questionnaire (FFQ) used to collect dietary data in this study only asked about three dietary sources of soy: tofu, miso, and soy-based vegetarian meat replacements.[10] This limited assessment of soy foods excludes some of the most commonly consumed soy products today, such as edamame, soy milk, soybeans, soy sauce, soy flour, and natto. Other studies on this subject conduct more holistic evaluations of soy intake by including far more soy products on their FFQs. By only assessing the intake of some soy products, this study may have inaccurately evaluated the true amount of soy products its participants were eating, thereby underestimating soy's protective effects against prostate cancer incidence and leading to an insignificant association between soy intake and prostate cancer risk.[10]

Another credible study that found soy consumption to be insignificantly associated with prostate cancer was a Japanese study conducted in 2000.[11] In this ecological study, the researchers investigated the connection between soy intake and cancer mortality. Dietary data for this project was collected from Japan's National Nutrition Survey (NNS). The NNS contained dietary information from around six thousand randomly selected households in Japan in the 1980s. After analysis, the findings from this study indicated that soy intake was not significantly associated with reducing men's risk for prostate cancer mortality.

It is important to note that this study looked at the impact of soy intake on prostate cancer mortality, not incidence or risk.[11] Recognizing this may alter the way we interpret the "insignificant association" found by this study because of our understanding of the mechanisms that soy isoflavones use to protect the body from prostate cancer. As previously mentioned, soy exerts its anti-cancer properties most strongly in the early stages of prostate cancer. We know that soy and soy products have been found to not be as protective against advanced stages of prostate cancer. Therefore, when evaluating the relationship between soy intake and prostate cancer mortality, which implies advanced stages of prostate cancer, it is not surprising that the association was found to be statistically insignificant. The findings from this study, while valid and worth mentioning, therefore cannot be directly compared to the other studies we have talked about so far, which discuss soy intake in relation to men's risk for prostate cancer.[11]

Appreciating the findings from these studies is important, but perhaps more important is recognizing that an insignificant association does not mean a negative or detrimental association. In other words, these studies found no harmful connection between soy intake and prostate cancer risk. Considering the many studies with evidence supporting the benefits of soy, it seems that the potential advantages of including soy in your daily diet may outweigh the potential neutral effects.

Aside from the potential anti-cancer perks of eating soy, this nutritious food also has many other health benefits. Namely, eating soy has been recognized by the Food and Drug Administration (FDA) and the American Heart Association (AHA) as an excellent way to reduce your risk for heart disease.[12] Soy contains all of the essential nutrients we need from a dietary protein source to stay healthy, which makes it a complete protein. Compared to animal proteins, soy is lower in both cholesterol and saturated fat, so replacing animal products with soy is an easy and effective way of lowering unhealthy blood cholesterol levels and protecting yourself from heart disease.[12] In fact, the FDA and the AHA both recommend that a diet that is low in saturated fats and cholesterol, which includes around 25 grams of soy per day, may reduce your risk for heart disease. It is worthwhile to note that the AHA specifically recommends eating soy protein whole, rather than taking an isoflavone supplement, as the maximum healing effects of soy can only be obtained from eating this food whole.

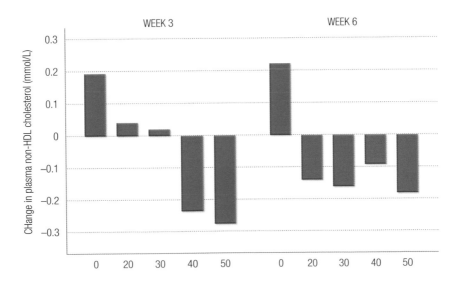

In a study published by the *American Journal of Clinical Nutrition*, researchers investigated how much soy people would need to eat to decrease their cholesterol levels.[13] High cholesterol is a recognized risk factor of heart disease. Therefore, the hope was that by decreasing men's cholesterol levels, soy intake would also by extension decrease their risk for heart disease. For this study, eighty-one men with hypercholesterolemia (high blood cholesterol levels) were recruited. Study participants were then randomly split into two groups, the intervention group and the control group. Men in the intervention group were given either 20, 30, 40, or 50 grams of soy per day; men in the control group were given the same conditions, but with animal protein. After a treatment period of six weeks, the participants' cholesterol levels were measured and compared. The figure on page 43, cropped directly from the article, illustrates the remarkable results of this experiment.[13] This graph displays participants' levels of unhealthy cholesterol over the course of this experiment ("Change in plasma non-HDL cholesterol") by their relative levels of soy intake ("Dietary ISP"). The first column in this bar graph represents the men who consumed only animal protein and ate no soy. This first column shows no significant change in cholesterol levels over time. Comparatively, participants at every level of soy intake displayed significantly lower cholesterol levels.[13] Put differently, at every level of soy protein intake, the men in the intervention group displayed significantly lower cholesterol levels than the men who ate animal protein. As men ate more soy, their cholesterol levels decreased in a proportional manner. Based on the results from this study, researchers concluded that eating as little as 20 grams of soy per day can significantly reduce your cholesterol levels and decrease your risk for heart disease![13]

In addition to reducing your chances for heart disease, soy has also been found to lower your risk for type 2 diabetes mellitus.[14] In 2008, a study followed 64,227 women in China to answer one question: How does eating soy products impact people's risk for type 2 diabetes? After nearly five years of evaluation, researchers found that the participants with the highest soy intake reduced their risk for type 2 diabetes by an impressive 47 percent when compared to those with the lowest soy intake. While soy consumption in general was associated with lowering the participants' risk for type 2 diabetes, soy milk and soy bean intake were specifically both significantly associated with reducing risk as well.[14] These findings add to the large body of evidence on the holistic health benefits of eating soy.

To ensure that you get the most bang for your buck when eating this powerful legume, here is a quick tip to maximizing the nutrient bioavailability in the soybeans you consume. Unprocessed soybeans have the highest content of isoflavones.[3, 15] In 2000, a study sampled fifty different soybean products to see which form of soy had the highest isoflavone concentrations. The results showed that any form of processing they analyzed, from heating to fermenting, significantly reduced the isoflavone concentration in the soybean products.[3] A second study found that refined, highly processed soy products may lose anywhere from 80 to 90 percent of their isoflavone content.[15] Therefore the most nutritionally effective way to add soybeans to your diet is in their raw form. A simple way to do this is through the tasty snack edamame. Edamame are soybeans that are still in their pods. Edamame are typically boiled or steamed, salted, and then popped out of their pods and eaten! This delicious snack is easy to make or buy, and even easier to love! When it comes to soybean products, those that are not highly processed, like tofu and soymilk, also have relatively high isoflavone content and should be prioritized over more processed forms of soybeans.[15]

One delicious way to enjoy your edamame is sautéed with some quick and easy savory flavors.

All in all, adding more soy to your daily diet could possibly reduce your risk for prostate cancer, heart disease, and type 2 diabetes. The soybean may be small, but it is mighty.

Sautéed Edamame

1 cup frozen edamame in pods

1½ tablespoons olive oil or sesame oil

2 cloves garlic, minced or pressed

Salt

Ground black pepper

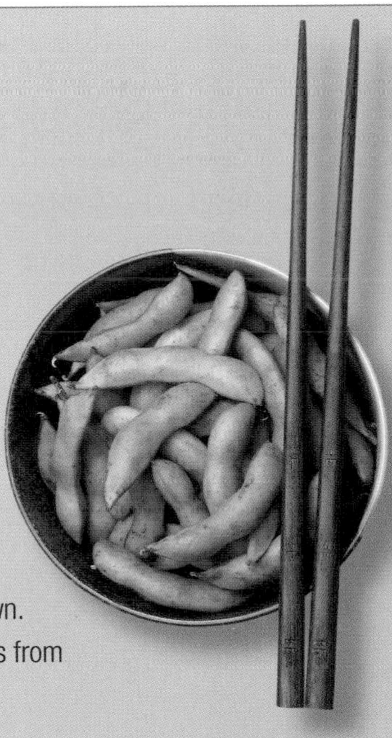

Fill a small or medium saucepan with water and bring to a boil over high heat. Add the edamame (in pods), boil for 3 to 4 minutes, then drain and rinse with cold water. Pat dry with a paper towel.

Put the oil and garlic in a skillet and place over high heat. Add the edamame and sauté until they begin to brown. Serve hot, or refrigerate and serve cold. Remove the beans from their pods and enjoy.

BIBLIOGRAPHY CHAPTER 4

1. "Soybean." *Britannica.com*. Accessed January 28, 2020. www.britannica.com/plant/soybean.

2. Roth, M. (2018). *Magic Bean: The Rise of Soy in America*. Lawrence, KS: University Press of Kansas.

3. Toda, T., Sakamoto, A., Takayanagi, T., Yokotsuka, K. (2000). Changes in isoflavone compositions of soybean foods during the cooking process. *Food Science and Technology Research*, 6(4):314–319. DOI:10.3136/fstr.6.314.

4. Pabich, M., and Materska, M. (2019). Biological effect of soy isoflavones in the prevention of civilization diseases. *Nutrients*, 11(7):E1660. DOI:10.3390/nu11071660.

5. Sivoˇnová, M.K., Kaplán, P., Tatarková, Z., Lichardusová, L., Dušenka, R., and Jureˇceková, J. (2019). Androgen receptor and soy isoflavones in prostate cancer (Review). *Molecular and Clinical Oncology*, 10(2):191–204. DOI: 10.3892/mco.2018.1792.

6. Jarred, R.A., Keikha, M., Dowling, C., McPherson, S.J., Clare, A.M., Husband, A.J., Pedersen, J.S., et al. (2002). Induction of apoptosis in low- to moderate-grade human prostate carcinoma by red clover-derived dietary isoflavones. *Cancer Epidemiology Biomarkers and Prevention*, 11(12):1689–1696. PMID:12496063.

7. Kurahashi, N., Iwasaki, M., Sasazuki, S., Otani, T., Inoue, M., and Tsugane, S. (2007). Soy product and isoflavone consumption in relation to prostate cancer in Japanese men. *Cancer Epidemiology, Biomarkers and Prevention*, 16(3):538–545. DOI:10.1158/1055-9965.EPI-06-0517.

8. Lee, M.M., Gomez, S.L., Chang, J.S., Wey, M., Wang, R.T., and Hsing, A.W. (2003). Soy and isoflavone consumption in relation to prostate cancer risk in China. *Cancer Epidemiology, Biomarkers and Prevention*, 12(7):665–668. PMID:12869409.

9. Sonoda, T., Nagata, Y., Mori, M., Miyanaga, N., Takashima, N., Okumura, K., Goto, K., et al. (2004). A case-control study of diet and prostate cancer in Japan: possible protective effects of traditional Japanese diet. *Cancer Science*, 95(3):238–242. DOI:10.1111/i.1349-7006.2004.tb02209.x.

10. Park, S.Y., Murphy, S.P., Wilkens, L.R., Henderson, B.E., and Kolonel, L.N. (2008). Legume and isoflavone intake and prostate cancer risk: The Multiethnic Cohort Study. *International Journal of Cancer*, 123():927–932. DOI: 10.1002/ijc.23594.

11. Nagata C. (2000). Ecological study of the association between soy product intake and mortality from cancer and heart disease in Japan. *International Journal of Epidemiology*, 29(5):832–836. DOI:10.1093/ije/29.5.832.

12. Erdman J.W., Jr. (2000). Soy protein and cardiovascular disease. A statement for healthcare professionals from the Nutrition Committee of the AHA. *Circulation*, 102(20):2555–2559. DOI:10.1161/01.CIR.102.20.2555.

13. Teixeira, S.R., Potter, S.M., Weigel, R., Hannum, S., Erdman, J.W., and Hasler, C.M. (2000). Effects of feeding 4 levels of soy protein for 3 and 6 weeks on

blood lipids and apolipoproteins in moderately hypercholesterolemic men. *American Journal of Clinical Nutrition*, 71(5):1077–1084. DOI:10.1093/ ajcn/71.5.1077.

14. Villegas, R., Gao, Y.T., Yang, G., Li, H.L., Elasy, T.A., Zheng, W., and Shu, X.O. (2008). Legume and soy food intake and the incidence of type 2 diabetes in the Shanghai Women's Health Study. *American Journal of Clinical Nutrition*, 87(1):162–167. DOI:10.1093/ajcn/87.1.162.

15. Messina, M. (2016). Soy and health update: Evaluation of the clinical and epidemiologic literature. *Nutrients*, 8(12):754. DOI:10.3390/nu8120754.

Additional Studies Not Detailed in the Chapter

16. Wu, Y., Zhang, L., Na, R., Xu, J., Xiong, Z., Zhang, N., Dai, W., Jiang, H., and Ding, Q. (2015). Plasma genistein and risk of prostate cancer in Chinese population. *International Urology and Nephrology*, 47(6):965–970. DOI:10.1007/ s11255-015-0981-5.

Based in China, this study examined the connection between plasma genistein (a prominent soy isoflavone) and prostate cancer risk. These researchers chose to evaluate plasma genistein because past studies have found this measure to be the result of soy intake. Therefore, by evaluating plasma genistein concentration and prostate cancer, these researchers are effectively measuring the impact of soy intake on prostate cancer risk. One hundred Chinese men were recruited for this project, forty-six of whom had prostate cancer. Plasma genistein concentrations were obtained via prostate biopsies. Results showed that the average plasma concentration of genistein were 513.0 ng/ml in participants with prostate cancer and 728.6 ng/ml in healthy participants. When comparing the significantly different average plasma genistein concentrations, findings indicated that a high concentration of plasma genistein was associated with a 69 percent reduction in prostate cancer risk. Based on their findings, these researchers speculated that high plasma concentration of genistein may be, in part, responsible for the lower prostate cancer incidence rates seen in Chinese populations. Moreover, these findings reinforce the hypothesis that soy isoflavones are protective against prostate cancer development.

17. Nagata, Y., Sugiyama, Y., Fukuta, F., Takayanagi, A., Masumori, N., Tsukamoto, T., Akasaka, H., et al. (2016). Relationship of serum levels and dietary intake of isoflavone, and the novel bacterium Slackia sp. strain NATTS with the risk of prostate cancer: a case-control study among Japanese men. *International Urology and Nephrology*, 48(9):1453–1460. DOI:10.1007/ s11255-016-1335-7.

Similar to the study led by Yishuo Wu, MD, (16), this study also investigated the connection between blood isoflavone levels and prostate cancer risk. These researchers compared the serum levels and dietary intakes of three major isoflavones (genistein, daidzein, and equol) of fifty-six Japanese men with prostate cancer with fifty-six controls. When comparing the highest to lowest serum levels, the highest serum levels of genistein, daidzein, and equol were associated with a respective 94 percent, 82 percent, and 48 percent decrease in prostate cancer risk. When comparing the highest to lowest dietary intakes, the highest intakes of genistein and daidzein were linked with a 14 percent and 20 percent decrease in prostate cancer risk, respectively. These findings suggest that high isoflavone serum concentrations may significantly reduce prostate cancer risk.

18. Jacobsen, B.K., Knutsen, S.F., and Fraser, G.E. (1998). Does high soy milk intake reduce prostate cancer incidence? The Adventist Health Study (United States). *Cancer Causes and Control*, 9(6):553–557. DOI:10.1023/a: 1008819500080.

    Using data from the Adventist Health Study, these researchers assessed the role of soy milk intake in men's risk for prostate cancer. Dietary data was collected from 12,394 men in California via food frequency questionnaires. During the follow-up period of up to sixteen years, 225 cases of prostate cancer were recorded. Findings from this study demonstrate a significant negative association between soy milk intake and prostate cancer risk. Participants who drank the most soy milk had a 70 percent lower chance of getting prostate cancer when compared to men who never drank soy milk.[1] Although soy milk intake was significantly associated with a reduced risk for localized prostate cancer, no association was found for advanced prostate cancer incidence. These findings reinforce the theory that soy products may reduce men's risk for localized prostate cancer incidence.

---

[1]The categories outlined on the FFQ for soy milk consumption were as follows: never, less than daily, once per day, greater than one time per day. It is important to note that only three men reported in the top category of soy milk consumption, so the confidence interval on this measure was very high. As such, any conclusions made on this measure are questionable, despite statistical significance. After merging the top two categories of soy milk intake (once daily and more than once daily), participants in the new highest category of soy milk intake had a 40 percent lower risk for prostate cancer incidence than those who never drank soy milk. This new percentage is still statistically significant and seems to be a more reasonable assessment of risk based on the data available.

Green Tea

Shifting gears away from foods with anti–prostate cancer properties, there are also equally impactful anti-cancer dietary choices in the form of beverages. With a reputation dating back to 2737 BCE China, green tea is known today as one of the healthiest drinks on Earth.[1] Tea is the second most consumed beverage worldwide, second only to water. More than two-thirds of the global population drink this historically embraced beverage.[2] Within the United States, tea can be found in nearly 80 percent of homes and on any given day more than 159 million people drink tea.[1] If you are one of the millions of Americans who drink tea every day, you may already know that in addition to being a delicious refreshment, green tea also has an abundance of health benefits. Throughout this chapter we will discuss these benefits, which include reducing your risk for prostate cancer and other common diseases.[2-8]

Before diving into the research on tea intake and disease prevention, let's start by understanding what tea is. Tea is made by steeping dried plant leaves in hot water. The most commonly consumed teas come from the leaves of the Camellia sinensis plant; these teas include green, black, and oolong.[2] Despite all coming from the same plant, these three teas are processed differently, which leads to each of them having

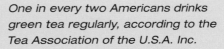

One in every two Americans drinks green tea regularly, according to the Tea Association of the U.S.A. Inc.

50%

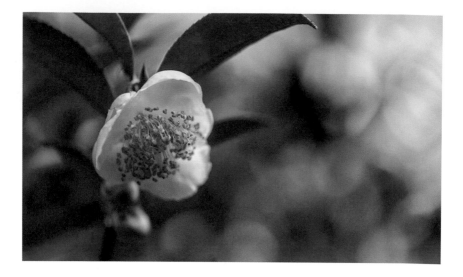

a unique chemical profile. One of the main ways teas differ from one another chemically is their flavonoid content.[3] Flavonoids are plant chemicals found in fruits, vegetables, and plants. When consumed, flavonoids can have a variety of healing effects. The most important flavonoids found in tea are polyphenolic catechins. The strong antioxidant properties of polyphenolic catechins have been identified as the part of tea that helps give this powerful drink its anti-cancer properties.[3] While black teas only have a 3 to 10 percent catechin content, green teas have a far more substantial catechin content of 30 to 42 percent. The difference in the amount of catechins found in these two teas makes green tea a far stronger antioxidant and consequently better at fighting cancer when compared to black tea.[3]

While we will cover the mechanisms that green tea uses to destroy cancer cells later in this chapter, knowing the major molecular differences between green and black tea is necessary in understanding why green tea's chemical composition makes it far better at fighting cancer. This understanding can also help explain why green tea, not black tea, has consistently displayed potent anti-cancer abilities in the current research on this topic and why it is the star of this chapter.

Speaking of research on this topic, we should start off by looking at a study that helped first establish the relationship between green tea consumption and men's risk for prostate cancer. This study was led by Norie Kurahashi, MD, from the National Cancer Center, Japan. For this study, Dr. Kurahashi utilized diet and lifestyle data from the Japan Public Health Center-based Prospective Study, which collected data from

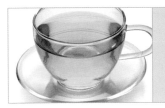

Men who drink the most green tea cut their prostate cancer risk nearly in half.

48%

more than 140,000 Japanese residents.[4] Looking specifically at the data provided by 49,920 eligible participants, Dr. Kurahashi and her team reviewed the lifestyle and dietary information collected from these men over a follow-up period of eleven to fourteen years.[4] Dr. Kurahashi and her colleagues may have expected to observe that an increase in green tea intake would help decrease men's risk for prostate cancer, but no one could have predicted how drastic this reduction would be. Although green tea intake was not found to be associated with localized prostate cancer risk, it was found to be significantly associated with men's risk for advanced prostate cancer. The results showed that the study participants who drank the most green tea had a 48 percent reduced risk for advanced prostate cancer incidence when compared to men who drank the least green tea.[4] By simply drinking green tea, these men were able to cut their risk for advanced prostate cancer nearly in half! Based on these findings, Dr. Kurahashi determined that green tea could significantly reduce men's risk for getting advanced prostate cancer.[4]

Dr. Kurahashi's extraordinary findings were echoed in a second, more recent study conducted in Vietnam. Headed by Van Dong Hoang, PhD, a graduate of the National Institute of Hygiene and Epidemiology, this study also aimed at defining the relationship between habitual tea intake and men's risk for prostate cancer incidence. For this study, Dr. Hoang recruited 253 Vietnamese men with prostate cancer and 419 healthy men, and compared their tea-drinking habits.[5] After

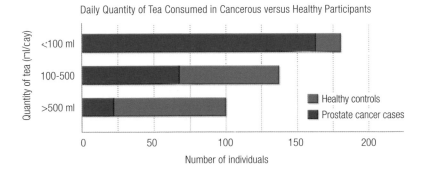

Daily Quantity of Tea Consumed in Cancerous versus Healthy Participants

reviewing the dietary information these men provided, Dr. Hoang found that in general the healthy participants drank far more green tea than the participants who had prostate cancer.

We created the graph above using the data from Dr. Hoang's study to illustrate the true impact of this research. This graph shows that the majority of the participants in this study who had prostate cancer drank less than 100 milliliters of green tea per day. After the 100 milliliters mark, the number of participants with cancer who drank tea every day dropped drastically. Comparatively, as tea intake increased, the number of healthy participants remained relatively high.

After further statistical analysis, it was discovered that at every mark above 100 milliliters per day, daily tea consumption was found to have preventive effects against prostate cancer. In fact, the results showed a significant, dose-dependent inverse association between green tea consumption and prostate cancer risk. Stated differently, the more tea participants drank, the lower their risk for prostate cancer was.[5] For example, participants drinking 100 to 500 milliliters per day of green tea had a 48 percent lower chance of getting prostate cancer, while those who drank over 500 milliliters per day were found to have a proportional increase in protection, with their risk being reduced by a grand total of 70 percent! These findings, as well as those from Dr. Kurahashi's study, point to the same conclusion: drinking green tea has the potential to significantly reduce your risk for getting prostate cancer.

Not only have scientific studies found that green tea can decrease your chances for getting prostate cancer, but research also indicates that green tea might be able to reverse cancer precursors in men who are at high risk for prostate cancer incidence.[6] In 2006, Saverio Bettuzzi, PhD, became interested in researching this topic. Dr. Bettuzzi is a professor of biochemistry and molecular biology in Italy. In addition to his tenure as a professor, Dr. Bettuzzi is well established in the world of cancer research, as he has been publishing impactful studies for the past forty years. Over the course of his four decades of research experience, Dr. Bettuzzi's work has in part focused on understanding how cancer progression can be blocked by green tea. Within this line of research, Dr. Bettuzzi decided to pursue a project aimed at investigating how green tea consumption would impact men with recognized precursors for prostate cancer. Dr. Bettuzzi chose to explore this topic because men diagnosed with prostate cancer precursors are at a much higher risk for developing prostate cancer.

Specifically, Dr. Bettuzzi looked at men with high-grade prostate intraepithelial neoplasia (HG-PIN).[6] While we are not going to delve into the details of HN-PIN, it is important to know that 30 percent of men who are diagnosed with HG-PIN develop prostate cancer within one year of diagnosis with this condition. HG-PIN is considered one of the most likely precursors of prostate cancer, making men with this condition a high-risk population for prostate cancer development.[4]

For his study, Dr. Bettuzzi recruited sixty participants who had been diagnosed with the prostate cancer precursor HG-PIN. Each participant was then randomly assigned to either the intervention group or the control group.[4] Men in the intervention group were given a pill with 200 milligrams of green tea catechin extracts three times a day. Men in the control group were given three identical placebo pills daily. After the participants followed this treatment plan for one year, Dr. Bettuzzi and his team collected the data on their prostate cancer incidence. They found that during the study period, only one prostate cancer tumor had been diagnosed in the intervention group (an incidence rate of 3 percent), while an astounding nine tumors had been diagnosed in the placebo group (an incidence rate of 30 percent).[6]

This significant difference in prostate cancer occurrence shows that the green tea treatment was able to prevent nine times the prostate cancer incidence in men who were previously at high risk for getting this disease. That means that the men in the treatment group had a 90 percent lower chance of being diagnosed with prostate cancer than the men in the control group. Let that statistic sink in for a minute.

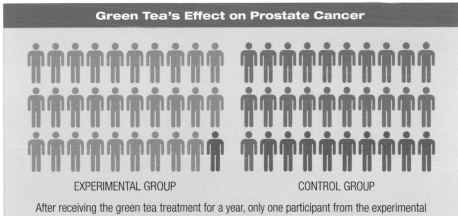

Green Tea's Effect on Prostate Cancer

EXPERIMENTAL GROUP   CONTROL GROUP

After receiving the green tea treatment for a year, only one participant from the experimental group was diagnosed with prostate cancer. Comparatively, nine participants from the control group were diagnosed with prostate cancer. The green tea treatment effectively prevented 90% of prostate cancer incidences in the experimental group compared to the control group.

In addition to reducing these men's risk for prostate cancer, another perk of the green tea treatment was that it had no negative side effects. Based on this significant decrease in prostate cancer incidence, Dr. Bettuzzi concluded that green tea can be an extremely effective and safe treatment option for the prevention of prostate cancer progression in men with prostate cancer precursors.[6]

Studies have demonstrated that green tea has the capacity to seriously reduce prostate cancer growth and development. Where exactly does this impressive cancer fighting ability come from? Well, green tea is packed with important nutrients, such as fluoride, iron, calcium, caffeine, and vitamin C, vitamin A, and vitamin K.[3] But, most importantly, green tea contains polyphenol catechins. Catechins are powerful antioxidants that make up 30 to 42 percent of green tea's nutrient profile. Antioxidants have strong anti-cancer powers, as we know from chapter 3, because they prevent oxidative damage that can lead to cells becoming cancerous.[3] While stopping oxidative damage is one of the most effective ways green tea catechins fight cancer, these anti-cancer warriors also use several other molecular processes to prevent prostate cancer. In a meta-analysis published in the acclaimed journal *Nutrition and Cancer,* the major catechins in green tea and the ways they prevent cancer were identified.[3] According to this article, there are four main catechin compounds responsible for green tea's anti-cancer properties: EGCG, EGC, ECG, and EC. While EGCG is the most studied of these compounds, all four have antioxidant capabilities and are most effective when consumed together in a cup of tea, as opposed to in an extract or as a supplement. These four compounds use several interconnected mechanisms to destroy prostate cancer cells, including blocking cancer cell replication, suppressing cancer growth, and promoting cancer cell death.[3] All of these

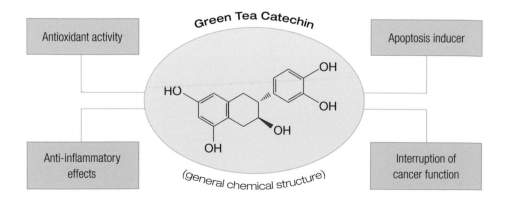

catechins and their various prevention mechanisms make green tea a powerful ally in the fight against prostate cancer.

One challenge when it comes to consuming this delicious beverage is ensuring that you are getting the biggest health bang for your buck. In his 2019 meta-analysis, Ping Dou, PhD, highlighted some of the barriers in developing green tea as a therapeutic agent, which range from nutrient bioavailability and stability to the relative efficacies of different strains of tea. So how can you make sure that you are getting the most health benefits possible from the green tea you consume? One way to do this is actually quite simple: pick the right tea.

After reading this chapter you may be motivated to go to your local grocery store and buy a box of green tea bags. Do not be tempted by the generic tea bags! Studies have found that a few specific varieties of green tea have significantly more catechin contents than others. By merely picking the right type of tea, you can boost the catechin content your body will get with each sip. These varieties, in order of catechin bioavailability, include sencha (Korean and Japanese), matcha, and gyokuro.[9]

How do we know that sencha is the best of the best? In a recent Polish study, researchers evaluated the qualities of twenty-seven unique varieties of green teas from six different countries to determine once and for all which type of tea had the highest catechin content. For each type of tea, the researchers collected three separate batches and then brewed three samples from each batch, resulting in a total of nine samples for each of the twenty-seven tea varieties. All of the brewed samples were then chemometrically analyzed for their catechin and metal content. The samples of green teas from Korea and Japan were found to contain the highest concentration of catechins, with the South Korean *jeoncha* (a type of sencha) being the richest in the catechin EGC and the Japanese sencha having the highest concentration of the catechin EGCG. Conversely, the green tea varieties from Nepal, India, and China were found to have the lowest concentrations of catechins.

Additionally, studies show that the best way to brew your tea to maximize its antioxidant capacity is by following two straightforward rules: longer and hotter. The ideal combination? Brew for five to ten minutes with near-boiling water.[10] Unfortunately, brewing tea for a period of this length can result in a slightly bitter flavor. An easy way to mitigate this is through the addition of healthy flavor enhancers, like lemon and honey. If you plan to store your tea, brewed tea should be refrigerated and consumed within a day or so to maintain the catechin content and antioxidant properties.[10] Finally, research has also indicated that loose-leaf tea can be reused up to six times and still provide antioxidant benefits, while bagged tea can only be reused up to two times. Both loose-leaf and bagged teas have been found to release the same total amount of catechins, so researchers have theorized that the bagged teas just release more catechins in their first few brews, while the loose-leaf teas release their antioxidants over the course of several brews.[10] This may be the result of the leaves in bagged teas being finely crushed before being bagged, which then leads to increased surface area on the leaves and faster nutrient release when compared to loose-leaf teas.

A physician-approved recipe for a nutritious green tea is a classic and delicious iced tea.

As if green tea's anti-cancer abilities were not enough, this incredible beverage also has numerous other health benefits. With positive effects impacting the span of the human body, it is no surprise that green tea is referred to as the healthiest drink on Earth. These healing effects include liver and cardiovascular protection, increased metabolism, decreased inflammation, bone fracture prevention, and anxiety reduction.[2]

One study, conducted in Japan, used data from the Ohsaki National Health Insurance Cohort Study to analyze the impact of tea consumption on people's risk for several cardiovascular diseases. Looking at lifestyle and dietary data from more than 40,500 participants that had been collected over an eleven-year period, these researchers made some impressive discoveries. After analysis, green tea intake was found to be significantly associated with reducing participants' risk for cardiovascular disease.[7] In fact, these researchers found that the study participants

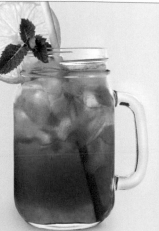

Chilled Sencha Tea

1 bag sencha tea for every 6 to 8 ounces water
Optional add-ins: lemon, honey, or mint leaves

Put the tea bag(s) in the bottom of a heatproof container and pour in hot water. Steep for 5 to 10 minutes, then remove the tea bag(s). Brewing for a longer time will result in a deeper, more bitter flavor. Cool to room temperature, then cover the container and refrigerate until chilled. Serve over ice and with the optional add-ins of your choice.

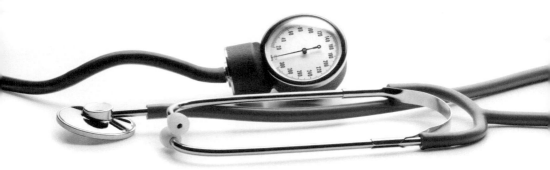

who drank five or more cups of green tea per day were able to reduce their risk of death from both heart attack and stroke by a significant 26 percent, relative to those who drank less than one cup per day.[7] In addition to reducing participants' risk for heart disease, this study also found that drinking green tea was associated with a general decrease in mortality due to all causes.

A second study that was published in 2018 found that drinking green tea can also significantly reduce your risk for getting another prevalent disease, type 2 diabetes.[8] For this study, researchers recruited 599 individuals with type 2 diabetes, and then found 599 age- and sex-matched healthy participants as controls. They then collected dietary data on the tea-drinking habits of all their participants, and compared the data between the healthy controls and the participants with type 2 diabetes. Generally, the healthy participants reported a higher consumption of tea in terms of the duration, frequency, and amount they drank. After adjusting for confounding variables, these researchers found that increased tea intake was significantly connected with a decreased risk for type 2 diabetes. Specifically, the people in this study who drank two or more cups of green tea per day had a 34 percent reduced risk for type 2 diabetes when compared to those drinking less than one cup a day.[8] Based on their findings, these researchers concluded that drinking green tea may be an effective method of reducing the risk of, and potentially even preventing, type 2 diabetes.

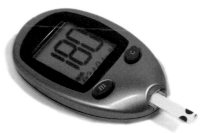

All studies considered, I think it is safe to conclude that green tea is a one-stop health shop. Masked as a tasty beverage, green tea is a health champion with the power to reduce your risk for prostate cancer and many other life-threatening diseases, including heart attacks, strokes, and type 2 diabetes.[1-8]

When thinking about maintaining a nutritious diet, it is natural to first think about the foods you eat. After reading this chapter, hopefully the beverages you choose to drink will also come to mind. The versatility and accessibility of green tea make it a seamless addition to any healthy lifestyle. Whether you are drinking your cup of green tea hot or iced, in the morning or in afternoon, at work or at home, you can always gain the rich health benefits of this delicious beverage.

BIBLIOGRAPHY CHAPTER 5

1. Tea Association of the U.S.A. Inc. "Tea Fact Sheet," page 2. Accessed December 20, 2021. www.teausa.com/teausa/images/Tea_Fact_2021.pdf.

2. Ping Dou, Q. (2019). Tea in health and disease. *Nutrients*, 11(4):929. DOI: 10.3390/nu11040929.

3. Connors, S.K., Chornokur, G., and Kumar, N.B. (2012). New insights into the mechanisms of green tea catechins in the chemoprevention of prostate cancer. *Nutrition and Cancer*, 64(1):4–22. DOI:10.1080/01635581.2012.630158.

4. Kurahashi, N., Sasazuki, S., Iwasaki, M., Inoue, M., Tsugane, S., and the JPHC Study Group (2008). Green tea consumption and prostate cancer risk in Japanese men: a prospective study. *American Journal of Epidemiology*, 167(1):71–77. DOI:10.1093/aje/kwm249.

5. Hoang, V.D., Lee, A.H., Pham, N.M., Xu, D., and Binns, C.W. (2016). Habitual tea consumption reduces prostate cancer risk in Vietnamese men: a case-control study. *Asian Pacific Journal of Cancer Prevention*, 17(11):4939–4944. DOI:10.22034/APJCP.2016.17.11.4939.

6. Bettuzzi, S., Brausi, M., Rizzi, F., Castagnetti, G., Peracchia, G., and Corti, A. (2006). Chemoprevention of human prostate cancer by oral administration of green tea catechins in volunteers with high-grade prostate intraepithelial neoplasia: a preliminary report from a one-year proof-of-principle study. *Cancer Research*, 66(2):1234–1240. DOI:10.1158/0008-5472.CAN-05-1145.

7. Kuriyama, S., Shimazu, T., Ohmori, K., Kikuchi, N., Nakaya, N., Nishino, Y., Tsubono, Y., et al. (2006). Green tea consumption and mortality due to cardiovascular disease, cancer, and all causes in Japan: the Ohsaki study. *JAMA*, 296(10):1255–1265. DOI:10.1001/jama.296.10.1255.

8. Nguyen, C.T., Lee, A.H., Pham, N.M., Do, V.V., Ngu, N.D., Tran, B.Q., and Binns, C. (2018). Habitual tea drinking associated with a lower risk of type 2 diabetes in Vietnamese adults. *Asia Pacific Journal of Clinical Nutrition*, 27(3):701–706. DOI:10.6133/apjcn.072017.08.

9. Koch, W., Kukula-Koch, W., Komsta, Ł., Marzec, Z., Szwerc, W., and Głowniak, K. (2018). Green tea quality evaluation based on its catechins and metals composition in combination with chemometric analysis. *Molecules*, 23(7):1689. DOI:10.3390/molecules23071689.

10. Pastoriza, S., Pérez-Burillo, S., and Rufián-Henares, J. (2017). How brewing parameters affect the healthy profile of tea. *Current Opinions in Food Science*, 14:7–12. DOI:10.1016/j.cofs.2016.12.001.

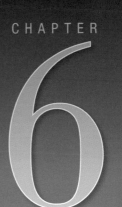

Foods to Avoid

he decision to make healthier food choices comes in two forms: the foods you choose to eat and the foods you choose not to eat. Just as eating more of certain foods can reduce your risk for prostate cancer, eating more of other foods can increase your risk for this disease. The consumption of three food items in particular have been found to notably increase your likelihood of getting prostate cancer. In this chapter we will be discussing the impact of eggs, dairy, and red meat on your prostate cancer risk.

Eggs

Although you may not be shocked that red meat and dairy products are "foods to avoid," you may have been surprised to see that eggs are too, so let's begin there. Eggs have long been promoted as an excellent source of protein and a healthy way to start your day. That being said, the integrity of eggs was recently called into question after several studies found that eating too many eggs is linked with increasing men's risk for prostate cancer. While research on this topic is rather limited, these studies are fairly unanimous in their conclusion on the risks of eating eggs in excess. One such study was conducted by Dagfinn Aune, PhD, MS. Dr. Aune has focused his decade of research in London on understanding how diet impacts diseases and mortality. Dr. Aune also worked for the World Cancer Research Fund, investigating nutrition and cancer risk on the global level. With his extensive experience in this area of research, Dr. Aune decided to be one of the first to tackle the relatively unexplored topic of eggs and prostate cancer risk.

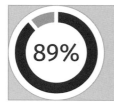

One study indicates that eating eggs in excess is associated with a significant 89% increased risk of prostate cancer.

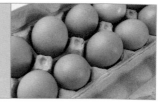

In 2009, Dr. Aune published an international study comparing dietary data from 3,539 men in Uruguay with cancer to 2,032 healthy men.[1] After following the dietary and lifestyle choices of these study participants for an average of nine years, Dr. Aune and his team found that high egg intake increased these men's risk not only for prostate cancer but also for colon, lung, and bladder cancers. In fact, they determined that the men with the highest egg intake had an increased risk for all cancers combined of 71 percent. Quantifying the impact of egg consumption on prostate cancer risk specifically, these researchers found that compared to those eating the smallest quantity of eggs, the study participants who ate the most eggs increased their prostate cancer risk by a staggering 89 percent.[1] These findings suggest that eating too many eggs can nearly double your risk for prostate cancer, while also indicating that eggs may increase your risk for other cancers as well.

Those are some astonishing statistics. They are so astonishing that you might be feeling a little doubtful about the validity of these findings. Despite these findings being statistically significant, meaning they are not due to chance, they still seem too extreme to be true, right? The scientific community was also skeptical after reading about this research, so a year after this study was published, Erin L. Richman, ScD, published a second study on the same topic. While Dr. Richman, from the Harvard T.H. Chan School of Public Health, was also interested in seeing the impact of eggs on prostate cancer, she chose to approach this topic from a different angle. Looking at men who had already been diagnosed with prostate cancer, Dr. Richman aimed to see how eating eggs would influence the progression or recurrence of these men's cancers.[2]

For her study, Dr. Richman followed the diets of nearly 1,300 men with prostate cancer for an average of two years. Participants were recruited from the Cancer of the Prostate Strategic Urologic Research Endeavor (CaPSURE). During her study, 127 of these men had some form of prostate cancer recurrence, ranging from cancer progression, to secondary treatments, and even to prostate cancer–related death.[2]

After analysis, Dr. Richman and her team found that the men who had consumed the most eggs during the study had a twofold increase in their risk of their prostate cancer recurring when compared to those who ate the fewest eggs. Put differently, the study participants who ate the most eggs increased the risk of their prostate cancer progressing or recurring by 102 percent.[2] On the flip side, the men who consumed one egg or less a week had no significant increase in their risk of their cancer advancing. These findings suggested to Dr. Richman and her team of researchers that post-diagnostic consumption of eggs may increase men's risk of their prostate cancer progressing and/or recurring.

So we have two studies, each exploring a different aspect of the connection between eggs and prostate cancer. The first study found that eggs may double your risk of getting prostate cancer, and the second study showed that if you already have prostate cancer, eggs may double the risk of your cancer progressing and recurring. These studies demonstrate the possible dangers of eating too many eggs, but you may still be unconvinced. If you are hungry for more, today is your lucky day because we saved the best study for last. What makes this next study the best? Well, the researchers in this third study recruited the largest number of participants, followed the participants for the longest period of time, and explored the impact of eggs on both prostate cancer risk *and* prostate cancer progression. Looking at 27,607 men over a fourteen-year period, these researchers analyzed the connection between egg intake and (1) men's risk of getting prostate cancer, and (2) men's risk of getting fatal cases of prostate cancer.[3] This study was able to complete both of these objectives by using the participants from the initial population (27,607 men) to assess the risk of getting prostate cancer and then looking at the subsect of these men who were diagnosed with prostate cancer over the course of this study to determine the lethality of those prostate cancer cases. During the fourteen-year follow-up period, 3,127 cases of prostate cancer were recorded. After analysis, results showed that the study participants who ate two and a half (or more) eggs per week increased their risk for lethal prostate cancer by 81 percent.[3]

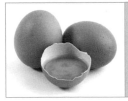

Eating 2.5+ eggs per week was associated with an 81% increased risk in fatal prostate cancer incidence.

81%

Conversely, the men who ate half an egg or less per week were not found to have a significantly elevated risk for lethal prostate cancer incidence. Looking at these results together, these researchers determined that eating too many eggs may increase men's risk for developing a deadly form of prostate cancer. This conclusion supports the findings from the two previous studies, by showing that eating too many eggs can both increase your risk of getting prostate cancer and increase your risk of cancer progression in the form of cancer-related death.[3]

What is it about eggs that could make them so dangerous for prostate health? Eggs are a rich source of dietary choline and cholesterol.[3] Both choline and cholesterol are essential nutrients, meaning your body needs them to survive.

While the majority of the choline your body needs to function has to be obtained from your diet, your body naturally produces all the healthy cholesterol you need to survive. This means that although it is important to find a modest dietary source of choline, dietary cholesterol is unnecessary and can even be dangerous. Research has shown that choline and cholesterol are highly concentrated in prostate cancer cells and that blood with higher concentrations of these nutrients is linked to an increased risk for advanced prostate cancer.[3] Furthermore, prostate cancer cells need choline to grow and multiply, and have been found to have a greater uptake of choline in comparison to

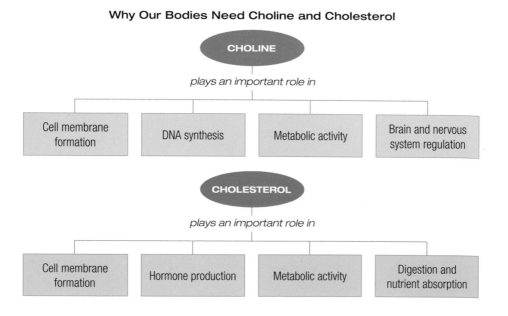

Why Our Bodies Need Choline and Cholesterol

CHOLINE

plays an important role in

| Cell membrane formation | DNA synthesis | Metabolic activity | Brain and nervous system regulation |

CHOLESTEROL

plays an important role in

| Cell membrane formation | Hormone production | Metabolic activity | Digestion and nutrient absorption |

healthy cells.[3] So, although a moderate intake of foods high in choline and cholesterol (like eggs) can be healthy, an excess of these foods can actually do your body more harm than good.

More research needs to be done before a conclusive recommendation can be made on a healthy quantity of eggs to consume, but for now one thing is clear. The limited current research on the relationship between eggs and prostate cancer generally points in the same direction: eating too many eggs may increase your risk for prostate cancer.

Dairy

Moving on to the second item in our "foods-to-avoid" trifecta—got milk? Unlike the limited body of research on eggs and prostate cancer, the exploration of dairy on men's risk for prostate cancer incidence is far more extensive and spans decades of scientific study. Research on this topic has by and large landed on the same conclusion: consuming dairy, especially high-fat dairy products, can potentially increase your risk of getting prostate cancer.

Let's jump right into this large body of work with a study led by June M. Chan, ScD, a Harvard graduate and current professor at the University of California San Francisco (UCSF) School of Medicine. Dr. Chan chose to focus her research on exploring the effects of diet, exercise, hormones, and genetics on prostate cancer incidence and progression. The goal of Dr. Chan's work over the last few decades has been to identify modifiable lifestyle risk factors for prostate cancer and help men create and integrate cancer risk-reducing strategies into their lives. With more than one hundred studies published on this area of research, Dr. Chan is truly an expert in this field. As such, Dr. Chan's study on the relationship between dairy and prostate cancer risk is an excellent place to start our journey. Using data from more than twenty thousand participants in the Physicians' Health Study, Dr. Chan's prospective study spanned eleven years of investigation.[4] Men who participated in this study completed dietary questionnaires to establish their dairy

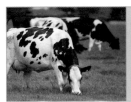

In a study with over 20,000 participants, dairy intake was found to increase the risk of prostate cancer by up to 34%.

34%

intake. After analyzing the men's responses to these questionnaires, Dr. Chan and her team found that dairy intake was in fact associated with increasing men's risk for prostate cancer. Specifically, Dr. Chan's findings showed that the men who consumed two and a half (or more) servings of dairy products per day had a 34 percent higher risk of getting prostate cancer[4] when compared to the men who consumed one-half (or fewer) servings per day. Based on her findings, Dr. Chan deduced that high dairy intake may increase men's risk for prostate cancer.

Dr. Chan's noteworthy findings were echoed a few years later by a European study that also aimed to determine the connection between dairy and prostate cancer risk. Although both studies explored the same topic, this newer European study recruited over seven times the number of participants. With dietary data collected from an impressive 142,251 men in the European Prospective Investigation into Cancer and Nutrition (EPIC), this is one of the largest studies conducted on the subject to date.[5] During the study's follow-up period of an average of 8.7 years, nearly three thousand cases of prostate cancer were recorded. Results revealed that the study participants who consumed the most dairy protein had a 22 percent higher risk for prostate cancer than those who ate the least dairy protein. Furthermore, participants who increased their dairy protein intake by 35 grams per day increased their prostate cancer risk to 32 percent.[5] In other words, upping their dairy protein intake by 35 grams per day increased their risk for prostate cancer from 22 percent to a shocking 32 percent. This association was particularly pronounced for advanced cases of prostate cancer.[5] These study findings further reinforced the theory that dairy products may increase your risk for getting prostate cancer, and specifically getting advanced forms of prostate cancer.

The current research on this topic is generally homogeneous in finding that dairy may increase your risk for prostate cancer. An interesting subsection of this research worth mentioning are the studies that explore the effects of the different levels of milk's fat content on prostate cancer risk. Specifically, several studies over the years have compared the relative impacts of low-fat versus whole milk on prostate cancer risks.

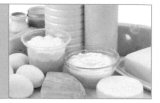

32%

A high intake of dairy was closely associated with a 32% increase in prostate cancer risk.

One of these studies was led by David Tat, a graduate of Duke University School of Medicine and an accomplished researcher in the UCSF Department of Urology. The purpose of Dr. Tat's study, which was published in the journal *The Prostate* in 2018, was to evaluate the relative associations between men's risk for prostate cancer recurrence and whole milk, low-fat milk, high-fat dairy products, and low-fat dairy products.[6] To accomplish this goal, Dr. Tat recruited 1,334 study participants with prostate cancer and then evaluated their diets.[6] Dietary data was collected from these men via food frequency questionnaires over an average of eight years.

Dr. Tat's findings were extraordinary. On one hand, the results indicated that men who consumed more than four servings of whole milk per week had a 73 percent higher chance of their prostate cancer progressing and/or recurring when compared to those who consumed three servings or less per month. On the other hand, the results also showed that the consumption of low-fat milk and other low-fat dairy products was not significantly connected to prostate cancer recurrence in participants.[6] These findings are intriguing because while whole milk was strongly linked with increasing men's risk for prostate cancer recurrence, low-fat milk and dairy products were not associated at all. Based on these results, Dr. Tat and his team concluded their article by recommending that men should choose non- or low-fat dairy options to avoid the potential prostate cancer–related risks that may be associated with dairy products that have higher fat content.

Dr. Tat is not alone in his findings. Another study looked at the diets of more than twenty thousand men for twenty-eight years to investigate the same topic.[7] In this second study, the researchers explored the connection between total dairy intake, low-fat milk intake, and whole milk intake in relation to prostate cancer risk. Due

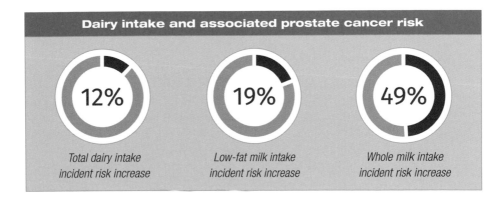

Dairy intake and associated prostate cancer risk

12%	19%	49%
Total dairy intake incident risk increase	Low-fat milk intake incident risk increase	Whole milk intake incident risk increase

to the longevity of this study, these researchers were actually able to conduct two related analyses. The first analysis looked at the connection between dairy intake and men's risk for getting prostate cancer, while the second analysis looked at the association between dairy intake and prostate cancer–related death (referred to in the literature as a survival analysis).[7] The results from the first analysis showed that (1) overall dairy intake was associated with an increase in prostate cancer risk, and (2) low-fat milk was linked with early-stage, non-aggressive prostate cancer incidence. Perhaps most importantly, the second analysis revealed that whole milk was significantly associated with the risk for fatal prostate cancer incidence. In fact, the participants with the highest intake of whole milk increased their risk for fatal prostate cancer by 49 percent.[7] Moreover, in the survival analysis the highest whole milk consumption was associated with a 117 percent increased risk in progression of all prostate cancer incidence to fatal prostate cancer post-diagnosis (in comparison to the lowest whole milk intake). Therefore, high whole milk consumption not only increased these men's risk for getting prostate cancer in the first place but also notably increased their risk of dying from prostate cancer as well.[7] These findings support the role of dairy intake, with a strong emphasis on whole milk, in increasing men's risk for prostate cancer incidence and prostate cancer–related mortality.

At this point, we've established that overall dairy intake, and specifically whole milk and high-fat dairy products, is associated with increasing men's risk for prostate cancer. As usual, we won't leave you guessing why dairy is potentially harmful to your prostate. Two mechanisms have been suggested for why dairy promotes prostate cancer, and both are related to dairy's nutrient content. Dairy is an excellent source of calcium and protein, both of which are essential nutrients for our bodies.[4] While dairy is a good dietary source of these nutrients, much like with eggs, too much of a good thing can end up being a bad thing. Firstly, high calcium concentrations can lead to the suppression of an active form of vitamin D.[4] Studies have found that vitamin D has important anti-tumor effects on human prostatic cells, so when it is inactivated prostate cells are more susceptible to becoming cancerous. In other words, when you eat too much dairy, the high calcium levels in your body block vitamin D, and without vitamin D it is harder to protect your prostate cells from becoming cancerous.[4]

The second mechanism dairy products may use to promote prostate cancer development can be traced back to dairy's high protein

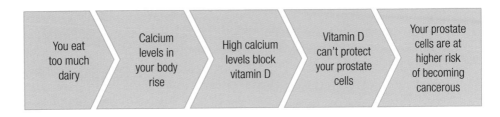

content. When you eat too much dairy, the high protein levels from this food can lead to the increase of a hormone called insulin-like growth factor 1 (IGF-1) in your body.[4] Studies have found that elevated concentrations of IGF-1 can be linked with a heightened risk for prostate cancer and an increased likelihood of prostate cancer progression.[4] Understanding these two mechanisms is important because they help explain why too much dairy can be damaging to your prostate health.

Red and Processed Meat

It's no secret that red meat is bad for you, but just how bad is it? For starters, in 2015 a published report from the International Agency for Research on Cancer (IARC), a branch of the World Health Organization, classified red and processed meats as carcinogens.[8] Carcinogens are substances that cause cancer. In their report, the IARC also separately recognized that red and processed meats directly increase men's risk for prostate cancer.[9]

As a division within the World Health Organization, the IARC would not make statements this bold unless they had been thoroughly researched. You should know that for their 2015 report on red and processed meats, the IARC recruited twenty-two of the leading cancer researchers from around the world. The conclusions these scientists reported were based on their evaluations of more than eight hundred studies on the topic of the carcinogenicity of red and processed meats. As defined by the IARC, processed meats include hot dogs, ham, bacon, sausage, and certain deli meats. The potentially health-hazardous forms of "processing" meats include salting, curing, fermenting, and smoking. Forms of red meat identified by the IARC as harmful include beef, pork, lamb, and goat. Finally, in addition to increasing men's risk for prostate cancer, these scientists also determined that eating red meat increases people's risk of colorectal and pancreatic cancer as well.

In 2018, a global study was conducted in 172 countries to determine the true extent of damage red meat can have on your prostate.[9]

To complete this study, data on the total meat intake and the prostate cancer incidence rates were collected from each of the 172 sample countries. Findings from this study surpassed everyone's expectations. Firstly, the results showed that total meat intake was strongly associated with increased prostate cancer incidence worldwide. Secondly, on the worldwide level, total meat intake was found to be an independent predictor of prostate cancer incidence.[9] In other words, across the globe, the amount of meat you eat was found to be its own predictor of your risk for prostate cancer, in the same way that genetics and age are independent predictors for this disease. The graph below, cropped directly from this article, displays the connection between meat intake and prostate cancer incidence by country. Each dot on this graph represents one of the 172 countries in this study. These dots are plotted along two axes, with the X axis displaying the total amount of meat consumed in a country and the Y axis displaying the number of recorded prostate cancer cases in that same country. As you can see, when a country's meat intake is low, their prostate cancer incidence is low as well. As meat intake rises, so does prostate cancer incidence in a linear fashion, with the countries that consume the largest quantities of meat having the highest rates of prostate cancer incidence.

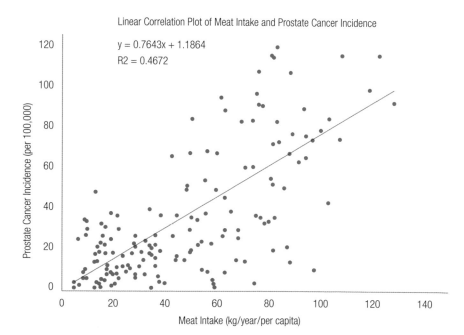

Linear Correlation Plot of Meat Intake and Prostate Cancer Incidence

$y = 0.7643x + 1.1864$
$R2 = 0.4672$

Furthermore, this study found that meat consumption was one of the major determinants of country-by-country variation in prostate cancer risk.[9] Put differently, eating meat is one of the main reasons some countries have far more prostate cancer cases and others have far less. To fully understand the weight of this statement, we need to go back to chapter 1 and look at the figure on page 4. This graph, which is cropped from the 2018 Global Cancer Statistics report, outlines the remarkably uneven distribution of prostate cancer cases around the world. The fact that this international study of meat and prostate cancer found that meat consumption was one of the main reasons for this variation is a strong statement, to say the least. This statement seriously reinforces the current leading theory on prostate cancer incidence, that lifestyle and your daily dietary choices can actually make a significant difference when it comes to your risk for getting this devastating disease.

So what is it about red and/or processed meats that makes them so incredibly detrimental to prostate health? Red meat is such an incredibly powerful carcinogen for many reasons, but for the sake of keeping this chapter concise we will briefly review only four of the major reasons. Firstly, when cooked at high temperatures, red and processed meats form heterocyclic amines.[9] Studies have found that heterocyclic amines are carcinogenic, which means they cause damage to your cells in ways that can lead to the cells becoming cancerous. Secondly, the preservatives that are added to processed meat, as well as the meat itself, produce N-nitroso compounds.[9] Like heterocyclic amines, N-nitroso compounds are known carcinogens. N-nitroso compounds mutate and damage your DNA in ways that can lead to your cells becoming cancerous. Thirdly, meat contains heme iron, which promotes the growth of carcinogenic compounds, such as the N-nitroso compounds just mentioned.[9] Finally, studies have found that meat may cause metabolic syndrome (MetS), which has been implicated in the development of prostate cancer.[9] These are only a handful of the molecular reasons why meat is such a potent carcinogen and strong promoter of prostate cancer.

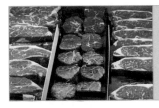

For every 10-gram increase in their meat intake, participants' risk for prostate cancer increased by 10%.

10%

Similar to the abundance of biochemical studies that examine why red meat increases your risk for prostate cancer, there are also many epidemiological studies on this topic. As a quick refresher, epidemiological studies attempt to explain how and why a disease occurs within a population by looking at specific risk factors that are associated with the disease. To start us off, let's look at an epidemiological study conducted by Rashmi Sinha, PhD, senior investigator, Metabolic Epidemiology Branch at the National Cancer Institute. At the National Cancer Institute, Dr. Sinha focuses her research on the connections between dietary choices and cancer risk. Within this area of work, Dr. Sinha decided to lead an epidemiological study on the connection between red meat and prostate cancer.[10] For this study, Dr. Sinha and her team analyzed dietary data from more than 175,000 men over a follow-up period of nine years, during which time 10,313 prostate cancer incidences were observed. Dr. Sinha and her team found that red and processed meats were significantly linked with increasing men's risk for both total and advanced prostate cancer incidence.[10] Participants with the highest red and processed meat intake increased their risk for advanced cases of prostate cancer by up to 32 percent when compared to those eating the least red and processed meat. What's more, the results from Dr. Sinha's study were dose dependent, indicating that for every 10-gram increase in intake of red processed meats, a participant's risk for advanced prostate cancer also increased by 10 percent.[10]

Dr. Sinha's findings are mirrored over and over again in current scientific literature. A second study on this topic, led by a professor and researcher at Imperial College London, evaluated the diets of nearly thirty thousand American men for a period of up to twenty-two years.[11] Over the course of the study, 1,338 cases of prostate cancer were recorded. After cross-analyzing the dietary data and prostate cancer incidence rates, the results exhibited a significant association between consuming very well-done meat and prostate cancer risk. As a matter of fact, the data from this study indicated that eating more than 10 grams of well-done meat per day was associated with a 42 percent increase in prostate cancer risk.[11]

In yet another study, researchers looked at the impact of red meat consumption after prostate cancer diagnosis.[12] In this Washington-based study, researchers collected dietary data via food frequency questionnaires from 971 men who had recently been diagnosed with prostate cancer over a seven-year period. After analysis, these researchers found that the men who consumed the most meat post-diagnosis had a 66 percent higher chance of having their prostate cancer recur in an advanced form. When the meat was cooked well done, this percentage was bumped up to a 74 percent increased chance for advanced cancer recurrence![12] These findings suggest that consuming red meat, especially when it is well done, may increase men's risk for prostate cancer recurrence in advanced, high-grade forms.

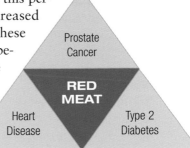

In addition to the damaging effects that meat, dairy, and eggs have on your prostate, eating these foods can also increase your risk for other chronic and life-threatening diseases.[13–16] In 2010, a meta-analysis on the health detriments of red meat was conducted with data from twenty studies and a combined total of 1,218,380 participants.[13] More precisely, this study aimed at understanding the influence of red and processed meat intake on coronary heart disease, stroke, and diabetes mellitus. Based on the data these researchers collected from the more than one million participants included in this study, the results showed significant associations between processed meats and both coronary heart disease and diabetes risk. When comparing the relative diets of the study participants, the findings indicated that the participants who consumed the most red and processed meats had a 42 percent higher risk of getting coronary heart disease (which can lead to a heart attack) and a 19 percent increased risk for diabetes onset.[13]

Another meta-analysis was conducted three years later to further explore the impact of red meat on type 2 diabetes mellitus risk.[14] This second meta-analysis included data from three American cohort studies and a combined total of more than two hundred thousand participants. Results from this analysis showed that both unprocessed and processed red meats were significantly linked with increasing participants' risk for getting type 2 diabetes. Specifically, these researchers found that a one serving per day increase of (1) unprocessed, (2) processed, and (3) total red meat intake was associated with a respective 12 percent, 32 percent, and 14 percent increased risk for type 2 diabetes.[14] Interestingly enough, when the participants in this study substituted one serving of the processed red meat with nuts, low-fat dairy, or whole grains every day, they were able to actually decrease their risk for diabetes by up to 35 percent![14]

So all in all, eating red and processed meat not only increases your risk for prostate cancer but it can also increase your risk for two other serious, life-threatening diseases: type 2 diabetes and coronary heart disease.[13–14]

As you may or may not have expected, red meat is not the only food item in this chapter that is a potential threat to your heart health. A meta-analysis published in 2019 looked at six prospective cohort studies to evaluate the effects that eating eggs can have on cardiovascular disease and general mortality.[15] After evaluating the diets of 29,651 study participants for an average of seventeen and a half years, these researchers discovered that eggs were significantly linked with increasing the study participants' risk for both heart disease and death in general. Findings indicated that each additional 300 milligrams of dietary cholesterol intake (in egg form) per day resulted in a 17 percent higher risk for cardiovascular disease and an 18 percent higher risk for mortality in general.[15] For reference, an average egg contains around 186 milligrams of cholesterol, meaning that the participants who experienced these observed increases in risk were eating only about an egg and a half per day. We've said it before and we'll say it again: eggs are a great example of how too much of a good thing can end up being a bad thing.

Finally, we've got milk. In a recent study, the association between dairy intake and Parkinson's disease risk was assessed.[16] To complete this study, researchers combined nine years' worth of dietary and disease incidence data from nearly sixty thousand men and more than seventy thousand women in the Cancer Prevention Study II Nutrition Cohort. During the span of this study, 388 cases of Parkinson's disease were identified in participants. After cross-referencing the dietary data with the incidence of Parkinson's disease, the findings showed that the men who ate the most dairy products increased their risk for Parkinson's by a shocking 80 percent.[16] Let's repeat that last sentence for emphasis. The men in this study who ate the most dairy had an 80 percent higher chance of getting Parkinson's disease than the men eating the least dairy. These findings suggest that in addition to increasing your risk for prostate cancer, high dairy intake can also significantly increase your risk for Parkinson's disease.[16]

If the thought of giving up cheeseburgers and omelets has your stomach in knots right now, don't worry—you aren't alone. No one is suggesting that you need to completely cut these foods out of your diet. By simply limiting your intake of eggs, dairy, and meat, you already give yourself a far better fighting chance against prostate cancer. One way to help limit your intake of these foods is by finding tasty replacements.

A study in 2016 found that when men substituted 30 grams per day of meat with non-meat alternatives, they were able to decrease their risk for prostate cancer progression by a significant 21 percent.[12] There are several healthy replacements for red meat and eggs, the best

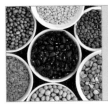

Start small: by substituting 30 grams per day of red meat with healthier proteins, you can reduce your risk for prostate cancer progression by up to 21%.

21%

of which seems to be soy (see chapter 4) because your body will get the protein it needs without the harmful consequences associated with meat and eggs. When it comes to dairy, substituting your high-fat dairy products with low-fat alternatives can be a simple and effective step in the right direction. The goal should be not to deprive yourself of the foods you love, but to instead focus on moderation and substitution as much as possible.

BIBLIOGRAPHY CHAPTER 6

1. Aune, D., De Stefani, E., Ronco, A.L., Boffetta, P., Deneo-Pellegrini, H., Acosta, G., and Mendilaharsu, M. (2009). Egg consumption and the risk of cancer: a multisite case-control study in Uruguay. *Asian Pacific Journal of Cancer Prevention*, 10(5):869–876. PMID:20104980.

2. Richman, E.L., Stampfer, M.J., Paciorek, A., Broering, J.M., Carroll, P.R., and Chan, J.M. (2010). Intakes of meat, fish, poultry, and eggs and risk of prostate cancer progression. *American Journal of Clinical Nutrition*, 91(3):712–721. DOI:10.3945/ajcn.2009.28471.

3. Richman, E.L., Kenfield, S.A., Stampfer, M.J., Giovannucci, E.L., and Chan, J.M. (2011). Egg, red meat, and poultry intake and risk of lethal prostate cancer in the prostate-specific antigen-era: incidence and survival. *Cancer Prevention Research*, 4(12):2110–2121. DOI:10.1158/1940-6207.CAPR-11-0354.

4. Chan, J.M., Stampfer, M.J., Ma, J., Gann, P.H., Gaziano, J.M., and Giovannucci, E.L. (2001). Dairy products, calcium, and prostate cancer risk in the Physicians' Health Study. *American Journal of Clinical Nutrition*, 74(4):549–554. DOI:10.1093/ajcn/74.4.549.

5. Allen, N.E., Key, T.J., Appleby, P.N., Travis, R.C., Roddam, A.W., and Tjønneland, A. (2008). Animal foods, protein, calcium and prostate cancer risk: the European Prospective Investigation into Cancer and Nutrition. *British Journal of Cancer*, 98(9):1574–1581. DOI:10.1038/sj.bjc.6604331.

6. Tat, D., Kenfield, S.A., Cowan, J.E., Broering, J.M., Carroll, P.R., Blarigan, E.L.V., and Chan, J.M. (2018). Milk and other dairy foods in relation to prostate cancer recurrence: Data from the cancer of the prostate strategic urologic research endeavor (CaPSURE™). *The Prostate*, 78(1):32–39. DOI:10.1002/pros.23441.

7. Song, Y., Chavarro, J.E., Cao, Y., Qiu, W., Mucci, L., Sesso, H.D., and Stampfer, M.J. (2013). Whole milk intake is associated with prostate cancer-specific mortality among U.S. male physicians. *The Journal of Nutrition*, 143(2):189–196. DOI:10.3945/jn.112.168484.

8. Bouvard, V., Loomis, D., Guyton, K.Z., Grosse, Y., Ghissassi, F.E., Benbrahim-Tallaa, L., Guha, N., et al. (2015). Carcinogenicity of consumption of red and processed meat. *The Lancet Oncology*, 16(16):1599–1600. DOI:10.1016/S1470-2045(15)00444-1.

9. You, W., and Henneberg, M. (2018). Prostate cancer incidence is correlated to total meat intake—a cross-national ecologic analysis of 172 countries. *Asian Pacific Journal of Cancer Prevention*, 19(8):2229–2239. DOI:10.22034/APJCP.2018.19.8.2229.

10. Sinha, R. Park, Y., Graubard, B.I., Leitzmann, M.F., Hollenbeck, A., Schatzkin, A., and Cross, A.J. (2009). Meat and meat-related compounds and risk of prostate cancer in a large prospective cohort study in the United States. *American Journal of Epidemiology*, 170(9):1165–1177. DOI:10.1093/aje/kwp280.

11. Cross, A.J., Peters, U., Kirsh, V.A., Andriole, G.L., Reding, D., Hayes, R.B., and Sinha, R. (2005). A prospective study of meat and meat mutagens and prostate cancer risk. *Cancer Research*, 65(24):11779–11784. DOI:10.1158/0008-5472.CAN-05-2191.

12. Wilson, K.M., Mucci, L.A., Drake, B.F., Preston, M.A., Stampfer, M.J., Giovannucci, E., and Kibel, A.S. (2016). Meat, fish, poultry, and egg intake at diagnosis and risk of prostate cancer progression. *Cancer Prevention Research*, 9(12):933–941. DOI:10.1158/1940-6207.CAPR-16-0070.

13. Micha, R., Wallace, S.K., and Mozaffarian, D. (2010). Red and processed meat consumption and risk of incident coronary heart disease, stroke, and diabetes mellitus: a systematic review and meta-analysis. *Circulation*, 121(21): 2271–2283. DOI:10.1161/CIRCULATIONAHA.109.924977.

14. Pan, A., Sun, Q., Bernstein, A.M., Schulze, M.B., Manson, J.E., Willett, W.C., and Hu, F.B. (2011). Red meat consumption and risk of type 2 diabetes: 3 cohorts of US adults and an updated meta-analysis. *American Journal of Clinical Nutrition*, 94(4):1088–1096. DOI:10.3945/ajcn.111.018978.

15. Zhong, V.W., Van Horn, L., Cornelis, M.C., Wilkins, J.T., Ning, H., Carnethon, M.R., Greenland, P. (2019). Associations of dietary cholesterol or egg consumption with incident cardiovascular disease and mortality. *JAMA*, 321(11):1081–1095. DOI: 10.1001/jama.2019.1572.

16. Chen, H., O'Reilly, E., McCullough, M.L., Rodriguez, C., Schwarzschild, M.A., Calle, E.E., Thun, M.J., and Ascherio, A. (2007). Consumption of dairy products and risk of Parkinson's disease. *American Journal of Epidemiology*, 165(9):998–1006. DOI:10.1093/aje/kwk089.

Obesity, BMI, and Exercise

O besity in the United States is an epidemic of extreme proportions. To fully understand the severity and pervasiveness of the obesity epidemic in the United States, let's look to the Centers for Disease Control and Prevention (CDC). According to the latest data available from the CDC on obesity in the United States, 47.6 percent of American adults are either obese or severely obese, and an additional 31.8 percent are overweight.[1] These statistics were reported in the CDC's National Center for Health Statistics obesity report in 2017. What's more, considering the upward trend of obesity rates in the United States, it is safe to assume these numbers are even higher today.

Obesity rates in the United States have been rapidly increasing for decades and are now at an all-time high.[1] Based on the CDC's National Health and Nutrition Examination Survey annual reports, adult obesity rates have nearly doubled over the past thirty years.[1] The graph below displays the steadily increasing rates of obesity and

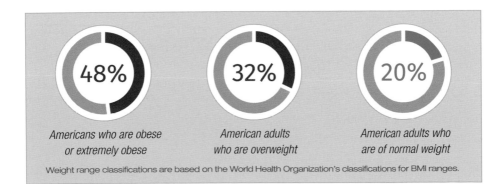

48%
Americans who are obese or extremely obese

32%
American adults who are overweight

20%
American adults who are of normal weight

Weight range classifications are based on the World Health Organization's classifications for BMI ranges.

severe obesity across all age groups (from twenty years old to sixty-plus years old) in the United States from the 1980s until 2016. In addition to noting the drastically increased rates of adult obesity over time, in their annual report the CDC also determined that obesity is associated with several serious, potentially life-threatening diseases. Due to these obesity-related health complications, when compared to individuals of normal weight, the CDC found that obese individuals spent an average of $1,500 more on medical costs in 2008.

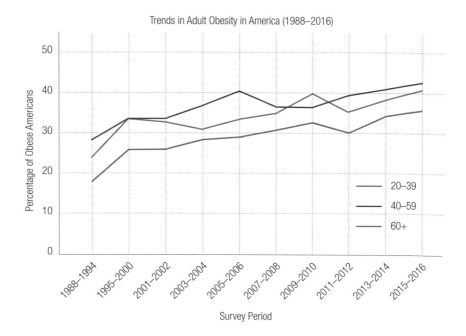

Trends in Adult Obesity in America (1988–2016)

Body mass index (BMI) is a common measurement used to classify weight categories. BMI is defined as weight (kilograms) divided by height (meters squared). When using this measurement in studies, most scientists follow the World Health Organization's classifications for BMI ranges, which are as follows:[2]

Underweight: BMI less than 18.5

Normal healthy weight: BMI between 18.5 and 24.9

Overweight : BMI between 25.0 and 29.9

Obese: BMI between 30.0 and 39.9

Morbidly obese: BMI 40.0 and above

The studies reviewed in this chapter all used BMI—the industry standard for measuring obesity—to evaluate the impact of obesity on men's risk for cancer and other potentially lifethreatening diseases.

Here to start off our journey into the world of obesity and cancer research is the late Eugenia Calle, MD, the former vice president of epidemiology at the American Cancer Society (ACS). Dr. Calle was a recognized and respected expert in the world of cancer research, especially when it came to the topics of nutrition, obesity, and cancer risk. Within her area of expertise, Dr. Calle chose to embark on a landmark study exploring the association between BMI and cancer mortality.[2] In pursuit of this objective, Dr. Calle and her team reviewed data from more than 900,000 American adults in the Cancer Prevention Study (CPS). Of the 900,000 adults in this study, approximately 404,500 were men and nearly 500,000 were women.

Over the course of the Cancer Prevention Study, which lasted 16 years, 32,303 male participants and 24,842 female participants died from cancer. After analyzing the data, Dr. Calle found that there was a significant connection between the cancer-related death rates and the participants' BMIs. In fact, the higher participants' BMIs were, the higher their risk of dying from cancer became. When compared to participants of normal weight, the men in the highest BMI category had a 52 percent greater chance of dying from cancer![2] While obesity was found to double these men's chance of dying from cancer in general, the researchers in this study also found that obesity was linked with increasing male and female death rates from several specific types of cancers. These specific forms of cancers included esophageal, colon, rectal, liver, gallbladder, pancreatic, and kidney. In men, BMI was also found to be significantly linked with increased death rates from stomach and prostate cancers.[2]

Based on these findings, which were published in the *New England Journal of Medicine*, Dr. Calle predicted that obesity may be the cause of 14 percent of the cancer-related deaths in American men and up to 20 percent of the cancer-related deaths in American women.[2] Something to keep in mind is that this study was conducted in 2003, when obesity rates were significantly lower than they are today. If this study were to be conducted again today, the percentage of obesity-related cancer death toll would undoubtedly be even more extreme.

So, by 2003, scientists already knew that obesity doubled men's risk of dying from cancer. The next step was to evaluate how much obesity impacted men's risk for specific cancers, like prostate cancer.

The data used in the study we just reviewed was collected from participants in the Cancer Prevention Study. The CPS was a long-term, large-scale study led by the American Cancer Society (ACS), which included participants from twenty-five states across the United States.[2] The goal of the CPS was to determine why people die from cancer. A decade after the CPS study ended, the ACS decided to start a second study. This new study was given a very original name: Cancer Prevention Study II (CPS II). In this new and improved study, more than one million participants were recruited from all fifty states, the District of Columbia, and Puerto Rico.[3] The data collected from participants in CPS II fueled another round of cancer research, this time on the topic of the specific cancer's causes and prevention.

Carmen Rodriguez, PhD, was one of the first researchers to tap into this new data gold mine. A senior epidemiologist at the American Cancer Society, Dr. Rodriguez published hundreds of scientific articles throughout her career. One of her most groundbreaking studies was published just one year before she passed away from adrenal cancer. For this study, Dr. Rodriguez evaluated the impact of obesity on men's risk for prostate cancer by reviewing data from nearly seventy thousand male participants in the CPS II.[3] Looking at participants' BMIs and weight fluctuations over time, Dr. Rodriguez and her team made two important discoveries.

The first discovery Dr. Rodriguez made was that having a high BMI significantly increased men's risk for getting high-grade, nonmetastatic and fatal prostate cancers.[3] When compared to men of normal weight, those with the highest BMIs increased their risk for these advanced forms of prostate cancer by 22 percent and their risk for lethal prostate cancer by 54 percent. In other words, the men in this study who were severely obese had double the chances of dying from prostate cancer. The second important observation was that the participants who lost eleven pounds or more over the first half of this study displayed a decrease in their risk for advanced prostate cancer by a whopping 42 percent.[3] So on one hand, Dr. Rodriguez found that obesity was significantly linked with increasing men's risk for getting aggressive and fatal prostate cancers. On the other hand, she also found that by simply losing weight, the men were able to markedly reduce nearly all of the weight-related increases in prostate cancer risks.[3] These findings substantiate the role of obesity in increasing men's risk for aggressive and fatal forms of prostate cancer, while also reinforcing the theory that weight loss may be an effective way of reducing this obesity-related cancer risk.

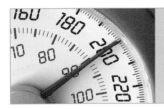

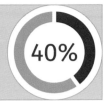

Study findings indicate that men with the highest BMIs had a 40% higher chance of getting a deadly form of prostate cancer.

40%

Another noteworthy study within this area of research was conducted in Sweden over a twenty-year follow-up period.[4] The goal of this Swedish study was to evaluate the connection between anthropometric measures and prostate cancer incidence and mortality. Anthropometric measures are quantitative human body measurements and proportions, such as height, weight, skinfold thickness, and BMI. To accomplish their research goal, these scientists analyzed the anthropometric measures of 135,006 Swedish construction workers for over two decades.[4] These measurements were collected via questionnaires by nurses when the participants first enrolled in the study. Throughout the study period, 2,368 cases of prostate cancer were recorded. After examining the data, the results showed that while BMI was associated with increasing men's risk of getting prostate cancer, it was even more strongly associated with increasing their risk of dying from prostate cancer. In fact, for each BMI category above normal, the risk for death from prostate cancer was significantly increased. In other words, as participants' weight increased, their excess risk for death from prostate cancer also significantly increased. When the data from participants in the highest and lowest BMI categories were compared, the participants with the highest BMIs had a 40 percent higher chance of getting lethal prostate cancer than those with the lowest BMIs.[4] Based on these results, this team of Swedish researchers speculated that body size (as measured by BMI) may be involved in the progression of prostate cancer from early stages to more aggressive, lethal stages.

While these scientists had three theories for why this could be, they knew one thing for sure: their findings showed that BMI is linked to increasing men's risk for prostate cancer incidence and strongly linked to increasing men's risk of dying from prostate cancer.

Looking at this Swedish study, Dr. Calle's research, and Dr. Rodriguez's work in isolation, the results are

OBESITY

Prostate cancer incidence

Prostate cancer mortality

certainly impactful. But when you look at these findings all together, a pattern begins to form. While obesity appears to be linked to men's risk for getting prostate cancer, each of these studies also highlights a potentially more concerning reality. While obesity is linked to prostate cancer incidence, it is even more strongly linked to prostate cancer mortality.[2-4] It seems that obesity is associated with increasing your risk for getting prostate cancer, and then significantly decreasing your chances of surviving this terrible disease.

When scientists realized this pattern in the data, they began hypothesizing why obesity seemed to explicitly increase men's risk for fatal prostate cancers. One of the leading theories today is that obesity promotes prostate cancer progression from early stages to lethal stages. This theory was made popular by a third CPS study, which hypothesized that the biological changes that occur within the human body as a result of obesity are also involved in prostate cancer progression.[5]

For this study, data was collected from both the CPS I cohort and CPS II cohort to analyze the connection between BMI and prostate cancer mortality. What did these researchers find? You guessed it! The results from this study showed a strong connection between obesity and prostate cancer mortality rates. Compared to participants of normal BMI, the obese participants had a 27 percent higher risk for dying from prostate cancer.[5] These findings indicate that decreased survival, not increased incidence, could be responsible for the link between BMI and prostate cancer. Put differently, these researchers believed that obesity did not increase men's risk for getting prostate cancer; instead it decreased their chances of surviving a prostate cancer diagnosis. These researchers theorized that this was because obesity, and specifically abdominal adiposity, contributes to prostate cancer progression through the bodily alterations that occur when humans become obese. Obesity causes changes in bodily hormone levels, increases insulin resistance, and can lead to hyperinsulinemia.[5] All three of these factors have also been found to be involved in prostate cancer progression. A second line of support for this theory is that obesity can reflect a poor diet and lack of exercise, both of which have been shown to change the human body in ways that can increase men's risk for getting prostate cancer.[4]

Although most of the studies we researched on this topic have largely found that obesity is associated with significantly increasing your risk for fatal prostate cancer incidence, there are also several studies that have not found a connection between BMI and prostate cancer risk.

One of these studies was led by Laurel Habel, PhD. As the associate director of Cancer Research for Kaiser Permanente Northern

California, Dr. Habel has been conducting research on the origins of cancer and cancer progression for over two decades. In this vein of work, Dr. Habel chose to explore the relationship between body size and prostate cancer risk.[6] To accomplish this goal, Dr. Habel analyzed anthropometric data from more than seventy thousand multiracial participants in the Kaiser Permanente Medical Care Program. During the study's nine-year follow-up period, a total of 2,079 cases of prostate cancer were recorded. Once the study findings had been analyzed, Dr. Habel and her team found no significant associations between weight, BMI, or a handful of other bodily measurements and prostate cancer risk in men. Simply put, the results showed no real connection between weight and men's risk for prostate cancer.[6]

Another large-scale study that found no association between obesity and prostate cancer was conducted in the Netherlands in 2000.[7] Looking at the anthropometric measures of 58,279 men for an average of six years, these researchers recorded 704 cases of prostate cancer. After adjusting for confounding variables (extra variables that the researchers did not account for), these researchers also found no clear connection between BMI and prostate cancer risk.[7] Furthermore, they did not see any significant associations between BMI and advanced prostate cancer risk. These findings, and Dr. Habel's findings, do not support the hypothesis that high BMIs may increase men's prostate cancer risk. That said, neither of these studies found that obesity can improve men's health or help reduce their risk of getting prostate cancer.

There is no easy explanation for why some studies have not found a significant connection between obesity and prostate cancer risk. Nonetheless, it is important to recognize that these studies exist. Discussing their valid findings is part of an objective analysis of the scientific studies on this subject. But, perhaps, it is more important to recognize that the vast majority of studies on this topic have found that obesity significantly increases your risk for prostate cancer incidence and even more strongly increases your risk for prostate cancer–related death. What's more, you would be hard-pressed to find a reliable scientific study that has found that obesity reduces your risk for prostate cancer.

There is powerful evidence that obesity can increase your risk for prostate cancer incidence, not to mention obesity is also a recognized risk factor for a multitude of other life-threatening conditions, including nine out of the ten leading causes of death in the United States.[8, 11–15]

In death toll order, the top ten causes of death in the United States are heart disease, cancer, unintentional injury, chronic lower respiratory disease, stroke, Alzheimer's disease, diabetes, influenza and pneumonia, suicide, and kidney disease. From these ten items, the only leading cause of death that obesity is not a risk factor for is, you guessed it, number three: unintentional injury.

We've already established that obesity significantly contributes to cancer incidence and mortality risk. Now, to better understand the other health risk factors associated with obesity, let's look at a study conducted in the early 2000s that evaluated the BMIs of American adults to see how BMI related to general disease incidence in the United States.[8]

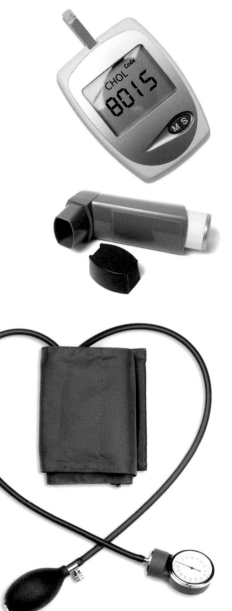

The primary goal of this study was to estimate the prevalence of obesity and diabetes among adults in the United States. The secondary objective of this study was to determine what other health risk factors, if any, can be related to obesity. To accomplish these objectives, these researchers harnessed data from the Behavioral Risk Factor Surveillance System (BRFSS). The BRFSS was a questionnaire distributed to 195,005 American adults that asked about personal behaviors that are considered to be risk factors for one or more of the ten leading causes of death in the United States. Behaviors included on the questionnaire ranged from anthropometric measures, like BMI, to self-reported incidences of diabetes, asthma, high blood pressure, and high cholesterol. Findings from this study indicated that being both overweight and obese were significantly associated with the following health risk factors: diabetes, high blood pressure, asthma, and high cholesterol. Compared to adults of normal weight (as classified by the World Health Organization's BMI ranges), severely obese adults had 7.37 times the risk for being diagnosed with diabetes, 2.72 times the risk of being diagnosed with asthma, 6.38 times the risk of having high blood pressure, and 1.88 times the risk of having high cholesterol. High blood pressure and high cholesterol are both known risk factors for cardiovascular disease. High blood pressure is also the main risk factor for stroke. Finally, high blood pressure and diabetes are both major risk factors for kidney disease. By significantly increasing these health risk factors, obesity can be effectively linked with increasing people's risk for heart disease, stroke, diabetes, and kidney disease.

Several studies have also found obesity to be a risk factor for depression, influenza, pneumonia, Alzheimer's disease, and dementia.[11-15]

All diseases considered, obesity may be one of the most dangerous threats to your health today. Luckily there is a foolproof way of reducing your obesity-related health risks. By living a healthier lifestyle, which consists of a combination of regular exercise and nutritious food choices, you can significantly decrease your weight and consequently any weight-related risks. The American Cancer Society's recommendations for a healthy lifestyle include both dietary choices and routine physical activity. But is it really essential to make healthy choices in both your daily diet and exercise practices?

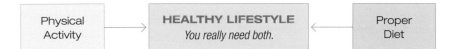

A study published in *Prostate* tackled this exact topic by evaluating the relative impacts of diet and exercise on men's ability to fight prostate cancer cells.[9] Participants in this study were split into three groups: (1) the men in group one followed the Pritikin program,[1] (2) the men in group two exercised for sixty minutes per day but made no dietary changes, and (3) the men in group three were sedentary and made no dietary changes. After participants followed their prescribed group's lifestyle regimen for fourteen years, their blood samples were collected and then put in culture dishes with human prostate cancer cells for three days. The goal of this experiment was to see which group's blood would destroy the most prostate cancer cells.[9]

After analysis, it was discovered that the blood from study participants in group one destroyed an average of 50 percent of the cancer cells in their culture dish. Group two blood was found to have destroyed 25 percent of the cancer cells on average. Finally, group three blood was able to destroy only 3 percent of the cancer cells.[9]

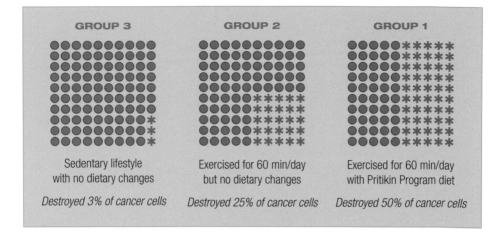

GROUP 3

Sedentary lifestyle
with no dietary changes

Destroyed 3% of cancer cells

GROUP 2

Exercised for 60 min/day
but no dietary changes

Destroyed 25% of cancer cells

GROUP 1

Exercised for 60 min/day
with Pritikin Program diet

Destroyed 50% of cancer cells

Let's begin by recognizing that the men from group three, who led sedentary lifestyles and made unhealthy food choices, had virtually no fighting chance against the cancerous cells. Comparatively the men in group one, who combined healthy practices in both exercise and diet, were capable of destroying half of their cancerous cells on average. That means that the blood from men living the healthiest lifestyle was able to destroy sixteen times more cancer cells than the blood from the men who made no lifestyle changes.[9]

Furthermore, the men who changed both their diets and exercise practices were able to kill off twice as many cancerous cells when compared to the men who only changed their exercising practices. Implementing regular exercise practices alone is undoubtedly impactful and can significantly improve your body's ability to fight diseases. That said, the combined effects of a healthy diet and regular exercise is the key to successfully giving your body its best fighting chance against obesity and cancer.[9]

Although we already discussed the American Cancer Society's healthy lifestyle guidelines in chapter 1, here's a quick recap. The ACS recommendations for a healthy diet include eating whole grains, at least 2 and a half cups of colorful vegetables every day, along with soy products and beans.[10] While the ACS guidelines discuss the healthy foods to include in your daily diet, they also emphasize that a healthy diet includes avoiding most animal products, especially red meat, eggs, and dairy. Lastly, when it comes to exercise, the ACS recommends an average of 20 minutes per day of physical activity.[10] Specifically, the ACS recommends 150 minutes of moderately intense physical activity

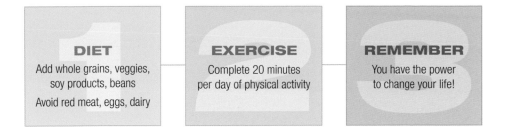

DIET	EXERCISE	REMEMBER
Add whole grains, veggies, soy products, beans Avoid red meat, eggs, dairy	Complete 20 minutes per day of physical activity	You have the power to change your life!

or 75 minutes of intense activity per week. In addition to these physical activity guidelines, they also recommend decreasing sitting time and sedentary lifestyle choices whenever possible.[10]

These recommendations are an excellent place to get yourself started on the track to a healthy weight, but they are still merely that—recommendations. They will not perfectly fit into every person's life. Find what works best for you and go from there. Being overweight may have the power to increase your risk for cancer, heart disease, stroke, and many other leading causes of death in America, but you have the power to control your weight. Take that power and make choices that will give your body the best fighting chance against prostate cancer and other life-threatening diseases.

BIBLIOGRAPHY CHAPTER 7

1. "Adult Obesity Facts." Centers for Disease Control and Prevention. Accessed March 4, 2020. www.cdc.gov/obesity/data/adult.html.

2. Calle, E.E., Rodriguez, C., Walker-Thurmond, K., and Thun, M.J. (2003). Overweight, obesity, and mortality from cancer in a prospectively studied cohort of U.S. adults. *The New England Journal of Medicine*, 348(17):1625–1638. DOI:10.1056/NEJMoa021423.

3. Rodriguez, C., Freedland, S.J., Deka, A., Jacobs, E.J., McCullough, M.L., Patel, A.V., Thun, M.J., and Calle, E.E. (2007). Body mass index, weight change, and risk of prostate cancer in the Cancer Prevention Study II Nutrition Cohort. *Cancer Epidemiology, Biomarkers and Prevention*, 16(1):63–69. DOI:10.1158/1055-9965.EPI-06-0754.

4. Andersson, S.O., Wolk, A., Bergström, R., Adami, H.O., Engholm, G., Englund, A., and Nyren, O. (1997). Body size and prostate cancer: a 20-year follow-up study among 135,006 Swedish construction workers. *Journal of the National Cancer Institute*, 895(5):385–389. DOI:10.1093/jnci/89.5.385.

5. Rodriguez, C., Patel, A.V., Calle, E.E., Jacobs, E.J., Chao, A., and Thun, M.J. (2001). Body mass index, height, and prostate cancer mortality in two large cohorts of adult men in the United States. *Cancer Epidemiology, Biomarkers and Prevention.* 10(4):345–353. PMID:11319175.

6. Habel, L.A., Van Den Eeden, S.K., and Friedman, G.D. (2000). Body size, age at shaving initiation, and prostate cancer in a large, multiracial cohort. *Prostate*, 43(2):136–143. DOI:10.1002/(sici)1097-0045(20000501)43:2<136::aid-pros8>3.0.co:2-l.

7. Schuurman, A.G., Goldbohm, R.A., Dorant, E., and Van Den Brandt, P.A. (2000). Anthropometry in relation to prostate cancer risk in the Netherlands Cohort Study. *American Journal of Epidemiology*, 151(6): 541-549. DOI: 10.1093/oxfordjournals.aje.a010241.

8. Mokdad, A.H., Ford, E.S., Bowman, B.A., Dietz, W.H., Vinicor, F., Bales, V.S., and Marks, J.S. (2003). Prevalence of obesity, diabetes, and obesity-related health risk factors, 2001. *JAMA*, 289(1):76–79. DOI:10.1001/jama.289.1.76.

9. Barnard, R.J., Ngo, T.H., Leung, P.S., Aronson, W.J., and Golding, L.A. (2003). A low-fat diet and/or strenuous exercise alters the IGF axis in vivo and reduces prostate tumor cell growth in vitro. *Prostate*, 56(3):201–206. DOI:10.1002/pros.10251.

10. Kushi, L.H., Doyle, C., McCullough, M., Rock, C.L., Demark-Wahnefried, W., Bandera, E.V., Gapstur, S., et al. (2012). American Cancer Society Guidelines on nutrition and physical activity for cancer prevention: reducing the risk of cancer with healthy food choices and physical activity. *CA: A Cancer Journal for Clinicians,* 62(1):30–67. DOI:10.3322/caac.20140.

Additional Studies Not Detailed in the Chapter

11. Luppino, F.S., de Wit, L.M., Bouvy, P.F., Stijnen, T., Cuijpers, P., Penninx, B.W.J.H., and Zitman, F.G. (2010). Overweight, obesity, and depression: a systematic review and meta-analysis of longitudinal studies. *JAMA Psychiatry,* 67(3):220–229. DOI:10.1001/archgenpsychiatry.2010.2.

    This meta-analysis conducted in 2010 compiled data from fifteen studies to determine the connection between BMI and depression. Studies selected for inclusion in this meta-analysis were all longitudinal evaluations of the bidirectional connection between depression and BMI. Looking at the bidirectional connection between depression and BMI means that these researchers explored the potential that not only does BMI impact depression, but that depression can also impact BMI. After adjustment, the results from this study showed a significant connection between obesity and the risk of depression onset. Compared to those with normal BMI, obese participants had a 57 percent higher risk for the onset of depression. Based on these findings, the researchers concluded that obesity may increase your risk for depression.

12. "Learn the Facts." American Foundation for Suicide Prevention. Accessed March 4, 2020. https://afsp.org/learn-the-facts.

    The American Foundation for Suicide Prevention states on their website that depression is the most common condition associated with suicide. Depression, especially when undiagnosed or untreated, increases suicide risk.

13. Santa-Olalla Peralta, P., Cortes-Garcia, M., Vicente-Herrero, M., Castrillo Villamandos, C., Arias-Bohigas, P., Pachon-del Amo, I., Sierra-Moros, M.J., Surveillance Group for New Influenza AVI, Control Team in Spain (2010). Risk factors for disease severity among hospitalised patients with 2009 pandemic influenza A (H1N1) in Spain, April–December 2009. *Eurosurveillance*, 15(38):pii 19667. DOI:10.2807/ese.15.38.19667-en.

In this article, researchers from Spain analyzed the characteristics of patients hospitalized after diagnosis with pandemic influenza A (H1N1) between April and December in 2009. During this period, 3,025 patients with H1N1 were hospitalized, 852 were placed in intensive care units, and 200 passed away. Based on the information collected from these patients, risk factors for H1N1 severity in adults were determined. Four factors in particular were found to be significant independent risk factors for worse disease outcomes: initiation time of antiviral therapy, BMI, presence of cardiovascular disease, and presence of chronic obstructive pulmonary disease. Specifically, morbid obesity was associated with a twofold increase in risk for H1N1 disease severity in adults. These findings indicate that obesity may play a role in increasing illness severity and even increase the risk of death in influenza patients.

14. Schreter, I., Kristian, P., and Tkacova, R. (2011). Obesity and risk of pneumonia in patients with influenza. *European Respiratory Journal*, 37(5):1298. DOI:10.1183/09031936.00188610.

Looking at a cohort of 158 patients hospitalized with pandemic influenza A (H1N1), these researchers evaluated the role of obesity in increasing patients' disease severity, by way of comorbidity contraction. Namely, this article investigated the impact of obesity on the development of pneumonia in patients hospitalized with H1N1. Of the patients evaluated, eighty were diagnosed with pneumonia. After analysis, BMI was found to be significantly associated with an increased risk for pneumonia. Compared to those of normal weight, patients with the highest BMIs had a 15 percent higher chance of contracting pneumonia. Although this study is limited by the small number of patients evaluated, these findings provide evidence that obesity may be an independent risk factor for influenza severity.

15. Whitmer, R.A., Gunderson, E.P., Quesenberry, C.P., Zhou, J., and Yaffe, K. (2007). Body mass index in midlife and risk of Alzheimer disease and vascular dementia. *Current Alzheimer Research*, 4(2):103–109. DOI:10.2174/15 6720507780362047.

Published in *Current Alzheimer Research*, this study evaluated the connection between BMI and the risk for Alzheimer's disease (AD) and vascular dementia (VaD). Looking at data from 10,136 participants for an average of thirty-six years, these researchers investigated the role of midlife BMI and later-life diagnosis with AD and VaD. Results showed that compared to those with normal midlife BMIs, participants who were obese in their midlives had over three times the risk for AD and five times the risk for VaD. Not only was obesity found to be a risk factor for these diseases, but simply being overweight was also found to be a significant risk factor as well. In fact, overweight participants were found to have a twofold increase in risk for both AD and VaD when compared to participants of normal weight. These findings support the hypothesis that high BMIs may increase people's risk for AD and VaD.

16. Freedland, S.J., Aronson, W.J., Kane, C.J., Presti, J.C., Amling, C.L., Elashoff, D., and Terris, M.K. (2004). Impact of obesity on biochemical control after radical prostatectomy for clinically localized prostate cancer: a report by the Shared Equal Access Regional Cancer Hospital database study group. *Journal of Clinical Oncology*, 22(3):446–453. DOI:10.1200/JCO.2004.04.181.

    Based in California, this study assessed the relationship between BMI and cancer progression after primary therapy.[1] In pursuit of this objective, these researchers followed 1,106 men diagnosed with prostate cancer who had undergone primary therapy for an average of four years. Over the follow-up period, participants were evaluated regularly for biochemical recurrence of their prostate cancer by means of PSA testing. Results showed that BMI was significantly associated with PSA failure (aka prostate cancer recurrence). Compared to men of normal BMI, those who were overweight had significantly higher risk of their prostate cancer recurring and those who were obese were at even higher risk. Based on their findings, these researchers determined that BMI was an independent predictor of PSA failure and, consequently, prostate cancer biochemical recurrence. Results from this study indicate that high BMI may significantly increase the risk of recurrence in men with prostate cancer.

17. Kenfield, S.A., Stampfer, M.J., Giovannucci, E., and Chan, J.M. (2011). Physical activity and survival after prostate cancer diagnosis in the Health Professionals Follow-Up Study. *Journal of Clinical Oncology*, 29(6):726–732. DOI:10.1200/JCO.2010.31.5226.

    Exploring the impact of exercise on prostate cancer progression, these researchers hoped to understand if physical activity would increase survival rates among men diagnosed with prostate cancer. After collecting data from 2,705 men diagnosed with prostate cancer over nearly a twenty-year period, these researchers discovered that men who were physically active significantly decreased their risk for both all-cause mortality and prostate cancer–related mortality. Participants who walked more than ninety minutes per week at a normal pace had a 46 percent lower mortality risk compared to men who went on shorter, slower walks. Furthermore, compared to men exercising for one hour or less per week, those who exercised vigorously for more than three hours per week decreased their risk of death from prostate cancer by 61 percent. By simply adding three hours of intensive exercise to their weeks, these men cut their risk for prostate cancer–related death by more than half. These findings provide support for exercise in decreasing men's risk for overall mortality and prostate cancer–related mortality.

18. Rimm, E.B., Stampfer, M.J., Giovannucci, E., Ascherio, A., Spiegelman, D., Colditz, G.A., and Willett, W.C. (1995). Body size and fat distribution as

---

[1]Primary therapy in this study refers to radical prostatectomy.

predictors of coronary heart disease among middle-aged and older US men. *American Journal of Epidemiology,* 141(12):1117–1127. DOI:10.1093/ox-fordjournals.aje.a117385.

The purpose of this study was to determine if BMI is an independent predictor of coronary heart disease (CHD). Over the study's follow-up period of three years, these researchers evaluated the BMIs of 29,122 men and recorded 420 incidences of CHD. Results displayed that BMI was, in fact, a significant and independent predictor of CHD in men under the age of sixty-five. Compared to men of normal BMI, those who were overweight had more than two times the risk for CHD, and those who were obese had over three times the risk for CHD. While there was still an association between BMI and CHD risk in men over sixty-five, the association was much weaker. Findings indicated that fat distribution, rather than BMI, was a stronger predictor of men's risk for CHD after the age of sixty-five. Based on these findings, it appears that high BMI may play a role in increasing and predicting men's risk for CHD.

19. Reynolds, G. (November 11, 2020). "How Exercise Might Affect Immunity to Lower Cancer Risk." *The New York Times.* www.nytimes.com/2020/11/11/well/move/how-exercise-might-affect-immunity-to-lower-cancer-risk.html.

This article analyzes and summarizes a recent study conducted in Stockholm, which explored the link between exercise, cancer growth, and white blood cells in animal models. For this study, researchers injected various types of cancer cells into mice, and then had some mice run and others remain sedentary for several weeks. After the intervention period, the mice's tumors were analyzed. Some of the running mice had reduced tumor growth when compared to the sedentary mice. These researchers then looked at the impact of exercise specifically on CD8+ T cells (immune cells that are effective in fighting cancer).

In their second experiment, these scientists blocked T cell action in the running mice with tumor cells. Although these mice were active, after several weeks their tumors still grew significantly. These findings, paired with the results from the first experiment, suggested that the CD8+ cells were somehow involved in preventing tumor growth, especially when combined with exercise.

In the third experiment, the scientists isolated the CD8+ T cells from the mice that had run and those that had not. They then injected one or the other variation of CD8+ T cells specifically into the mice that had been sedentary. The sedentary mice that received CD8+ T cells from the running mice were able to reduce tumor growth significantly better than those who had received the CD8+ T cells from the sedentary mice.

After analyzing the results of these three experiments together, these scientists wanted to determine why exercise seemed to impact the efficacy of CD8+ T cells in fighting tumors. In their fourth experiment, they drew blood from the running mice and sedentary mice and compared the two samples. The blood of the running mice was found to have more molecules related to fuel and metabolism, with a specifically high concentration of lactate. The scientists then took lactate and added it to CD8+ T cell mice samples. When they did this, the sample cells became more active and effective in fighting off cancerous cells.

Based on these findings, it was concluded that the lactate produced during exercise may help increase the efficacy of CD8+ T cells in destroying cancer cells. The findings from this study also indicate that the adaptive immune system, and specifically CD8+ T cells, is a critical aspect of exercise-related tumor suppression. This conclusion is preliminary and cannot be directly applied to humans, as it was determined using animal models. That said, like mice, humans produce excess lactate after exercising, but it is still uncertain if lactate impacts human CD8+ T cells in the same way as it does mice CD8+ T cells.

20. Rundqvist, H., Velic, P., Barbieri, L., Gameiro, P.A., Bargiela, D., Gojkovic, M., Mijwel, S., Reitzner, S.M., Wulliman, D., Ahlstedt, E., Ule, J., Ostman, A., and Johnson, R.S. (2020). Cytotoxic T-cells mediate exercise-induced reductions in tumor growth. *eLife, 9:*e59996. DOI:10.7554/eLife.59996.

This study aimed to determine how exercise impacts the immune system on a molecular level. The immune system uses cytotoxic T cells to identify and destroy cancer, preventing tumor growth. Data from the current study demonstrates that after acute exercise, mice muscles produced metabolites (lactate and TCA metabolites), which accumulated in their plasma and secondary lymphoid organs. This metabolite accumulation led to altered central carbon metabolism in CD8+ T cells, improving their anti-tumor effects. The parameters of this study are outlined in the article summary nineteen; additional details can be found below.

Flow cytometry was used during analysis to identify the molecular content of the mice blood samples. When comparing the samples from the exercising mice with the sedentary ones, only the CD8+ T cells were found to be significantly different (increased in running animals); no significant differences were found in the concentrations of intratumoral macrophages or neutrophils, CD4+, or NK cells.

During the second experiment, the mice were injected with an anti-CD8 antibody to reduce the number of CD8+ T cells in subjects; consequently tumor growth increased and long-term survival decreased. These findings demonstrated the efficacy of these T cells in tumor growth suppression.

Mass spectrometry was used to analyze the content of the mice's skeletal muscles and plasma after high intensity exercise. Findings showed reduced concentrations of glycolytic metabolites and increased TCA metabolites (citric acid, malic acid, and aKG) by two- to eightfold in both muscle and plasma samples. The biggest difference was in circulating lactate, with exercising mice having a much higher concentration of circulating lactate. This result was mimicked when analyzing samples from human subjects. When in the presence of lactate for seventy-two hours, CD8+ T cells displayed increased cytotoxicity against tumor cells. To confirm this finding, the researchers conducted another experiment in which mice were injected with daily infusions of 2 grams per kilogram of sodium L-lactate (mimicking the plasma lactate levels during intensive exercise), and their tumor growth was observed over time. Mice injected with the I3TC cell line (animal model of breast cancer) displayed reduced tumor growth, as did the mice injected with the colon adenocarcinoma MC38 cell line. Injections with lower concentrations of lactate did not impact tumor growth. These injections increased levels of CD4+ and CD8+ T cells, but decreased NK cell levels in subjects. The daily lactate injections were rendered ineffective when an anti-CD8 antibody was introduced. This indicates that the combined effect of lactate and CD8+ T cells was responsible for reducing tumor growth.

Other animal studies have found added pathways by which exercise reduces tumor growth, including decreasing inflammation, healthy weight maintenance, controlling endocrine hormone levels, altering tumor vascularization, improving immune function, and increasing levels of NK and CD8+ T cells.

21. Moore, S.C., Lee, I.M., Weiderpass, E., Campbell, P.T., Sampson, J.N., Kitahara, C.M., Keadle, S.K., et al. (2016). Association of leisure-time physical activity with risk of 26 types of cancer in 1.44 million adults. *JAMA Internal Medicine*, 176(6):816–825. DOI:10.1001/jamainternmed.2016.1548.

The objective of this meta-analysis was to determine the connection between physical activity and cancer incidence. A secondary objective was to see if this connection would vary based on body size and/or smoking status. Data for this meta-analysis was collected from twelve prospective cohort studies in the United States and Europe. In these studies, participants self-reported their physical activity levels, with each study falling between the years of 1987 and 2004. While data was collected from a total of 1.44 million participants, the participants ranged significantly in age (nineteen to ninety-eight years), cancer type, and activity level (moderate and vigorous intensity). During analysis, hazard ratios between high (ninetieth percentile) versus low (tenth percentile) levels of activity were used to determine association.

High levels of exercise were found to significantly lower the risk of thirteen out of twenty-six cancer types when compared with lower levels of exercise. These cancers include esophageal adenocarcinoma (42 percent reduced risk), liver (27 percent reduced risk), lung (26 percent reduced risk), kidney (23 percent reduced risk), gastric cardia (22 percent reduced risk), endometrial (21 percent reduced risk), myeloid leukemia (20 percent reduced risk), myeloma (17 percent reduced risk), colon (16 percent reduced risk), head and neck (15 percent reduced risk), rectal (87 percent reduced risk), bladder (13 percent reduced risk), and breast (10 percent reduced risk). After adjusting for BMI, the association between exercise and cancer incidence remained significant for ten of the thirteen cancers. Association remained fairly consistent between overweight, obese, and normal-weight participants, indicating that the benefits of exercise in reducing cancer risk persists regardless of body size. Smoking status only altered the association with lung cancer.

Finally, exercise was linked with a small increase in prostate cancer risk (5 percent increased risk) and malignant melanoma risk (27 percent increased risk). The modest associated increase in prostate cancer risk and exercise could be attributed to increased screening in men who exercise. The significant increase in melanoma risk could be attributed to the additional sun exposure associated with exercising outdoors.

Hypotheses listed in this study for the biological connection between exercise and reduced cancer risk include mediated hormonal systems (insulin, insulin-like growth factors, adipokines, and sex seroids), reduced inflammation and oxidative stress, and improved immune function.

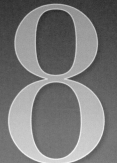

Screening for Prostate Cancer

 healthy lifestyle is the best way to reduce your risk for getting prostate cancer, and in some cases to prevent prostate cancer entirely. The foods you choose to eat, and those you choose not to eat, are powerful tools in the fight against this devastating disease, as is the physical activity you choose to incorporate into your everyday practices. That said, there is a third element in the "prevention lifestyle" that can be considered just as important as diet and exercise. This third element is routine screening.

In general, the American Cancer Society (ACS) recommends beginning discussions about your risk for prostate cancer with your primary care physician around the age of fifty.[1] The ACS one-sheet "Should I Be Tested for Prostate Cancer?" can be a helpful tool in determining what age you should begin consulting your primary care physician about your prostate. This resource provides broad recommendations based on your individual health profile, family history,

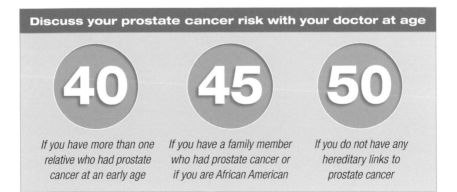

Discuss your prostate cancer risk with your doctor at age

40	45	50
If you have more than one relative who had prostate cancer at an early age	If you have a family member who had prostate cancer or if you are African American	If you do not have any hereditary links to prostate cancer

race, and personal preferences.[1] It is valuable to begin discussions about your prostate with your physician earlier, rather than later, especially if you have one or more of the factors that place you at a higher risk for this disease. An example of a factor that will undoubtedly place you at higher risk is genetics. Heredity is a strong contributor to your individual risk for prostate cancer incidence. In fact, if you have a family history of prostate cancer or are African American, the ACS recommends beginning discussing your prostate health with your physician by the time you turn forty-five, rather than fifty. If you have multiple family members who had prostate cancer before the age of sixty-five, you should consider having these conversations even earlier, when you are forty.[1]

While starting the prostate cancer conversation with your physician is invaluable, the next step in preventing this disease is equally significant: routine prostate check-ins. By and large, there are two forms of prostate check-ins: screening tests and diagnostic tests. The purpose of a screening test is to see if you have any of the signs or symptoms for a given disease. Screening tests can be conducted on a regular basis, as they are generally quick and easy procedures.[3] Diagnostic tests, on the other hand, are conducted to determine whether or not you actually have a given disease. Diagnostic tests can be more invasive and expensive, and are typically only conducted as a result of an abnormal screening test. Let's begin by first discussing prostate cancer screenings.

There are two forms of prostate cancer screenings: self-screenings and medical screenings.

Self-screenings are simple and can be done at home on a routine basis. Frequently conducting self-screenings could be helpful, as detecting prostate cancer early can quite literally be a lifesaver. If you are interested in adding self-screenings into your lifestyle practices but don't know where to start, have no fear! We have created an easy checklist for you with the signs and symptoms that Maurie Markman, MD, the president of Medicine and Science at the Cancer Treatment Centers of America, recommends you should look out for when conducting a self-screening for prostate cancer.

You can go through this quick four-item checklist regularly, but if you notice that you have any of these warning signs, you should contact your physician for a more advanced screening. That said, this checklist is not conclusive, so do not panic if you find yourself displaying any of these symptoms, as they can pertain to noncancerous prostate conditions as well. Moreover, a lack of symptoms does not

PROSTATE CANCER PREVENTION SELF-SCREENING CHECKLIST

Use this four-point checklist regularly to identify warning signs and symptoms of prostate cancer.

Your prostate is located near your bladder, with your urethra running through its center. Because of its location, prostate cancer symptoms may manifest in alterations in urinary patterns and tendencies.

○ Warning signs: frequent urination, weak urine flow, interrupted urine flow, painful urination, or blood in the urine.

Your prostate is responsible for creating the fluid that protects your sperm. When you ejaculate, this fluid combines with sperm to form semen.

○ Warning signs: finding blood in your semen, new-onset erectile dysfunction, or painful ejaculation.

In some prostate cancer cases the prostate can become enlarged.

○ Warning sign: discomfort while sitting, potentially caused by an enlarged prostate.

○ Some of the first signs of cancer to look for include unintentional weight loss, unusual coughing, swelling of the legs, and /or persistent back pain.

Disclaimer: *This checklist is not conclusive. If you have any of the listed symptoms, do not panic, as they may also be indicators of noncancerous prostate conditions. If you have one or more of the listed symptoms, contact your physician to schedule more advanced prostate cancer screening.*

rule out the existence of cancer, so routinely discussing your prostate health with your physician is still necessary.

In addition to personal screenings, another preventive measure you can consider, after discussing with your physician, is medical prostate cancer screening. Although we will outline your medical screening options here, please recognize that this outline is generalized and, as such, is not tailored to your specific situation, health profile, and medical history. This chapter can absolutely be used as a starting point for a prostate screening discussion with your primary care physician, but it should not be your end point. Talking about this information with your health care provider will enable you to understand how prostate cancer screenings relate to you. This will, in turn, help you and your physician create an informed, personalized health plan with which you are comfortable.[4, 5]

Currently, there are two common medical screening options: the prostate-specific antigen blood test and the digital rectal exam (DRE). Both of these options have benefits and drawbacks, so let's dive a little deeper.

Healthy prostate cells produce a small amount of a protein called prostate-specific antigen (PSA). The PSA protein is part of your body's normal production of semen. Although the PSA protein is typically found in semen, a small but significant amount can also be found in your blood.[3] As your blood PSA levels increase, so do your chances of currently having prostate cancer. During a PSA blood test, your physician is testing to see how high your blood concentration of PSA is. Your physician will then use this number to determine what your chances of currently having prostate cancer are. Blood PSA levels are measured in units of nanograms of protein per milliliter of blood (ng/mL).[3]

- PSA levels for men without prostate cancer are usually at or under 4 ng/mL.
- PSA levels between 4 to 10 ng/mL indicate a 25 percent chance of having prostate cancer.
- PSA levels above 10 signify over a 50 percent chance of having prostate cancer.

Before we go any further, let's make one thing clear. The PSA blood test is not a perfect science. Approximately 15 percent of men with normal blood PSA levels (less than 4 ng/mL) are still found to have prostate cancer if they complete a biopsy.[3] There are also incidences in which men with elevated PSA levels are found to not have prostate cancer after a biopsy is completed. These irregularities occur because, in addi-

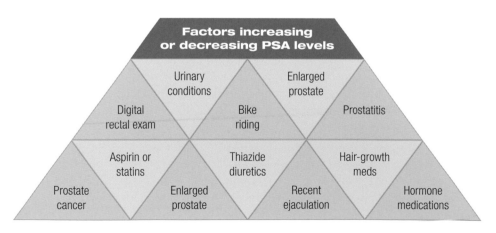

Factors increasing or decreasing PSA levels

Urinary conditions

Enlarged prostate

Digital rectal exam

Bike riding

Prostatitis

Aspirin or statins

Thiazide diuretics

Hair-growth meds

Prostate cancer

Enlarged prostate

Recent ejaculation

Hormone medications

tion to cancer, there are several other factors that have been known to increase PSA blood levels. Factors other than cancer that may also raise your PSA levels include noncancerous prostate conditions like prostatitis or an enlarged prostate, bike riding, recent ejaculation, hormone medications such as testosterone, and prostate-related medical procedures (that is, prostate biopsy and DRE).

At the same time, there are factors unrelated to cancer that may lower your PSA levels. Studies have found that some medications and herbal dietary supplements may lower your PSA levels, but findings from these studies are inconclusive. These factors include long-term use of aspirin, statins, thiazide diuretics, and the usage of certain medications for promoting hair growth, urinary conditions, and benign prostatic hyperplasia (enlarged prostate).[3]

All that said, the PSA blood test is a fairly accurate assessment of your chance of having prostate cancer and is the most commonly used screening method within health care. In fact, the United States Preventive Services Task Force (USPSTF) recognizes that PSA testing can have a small but significant impact in preventing prostate cancer–related death in men.[4]

The USPSTF is a nationally recognized volunteer panel of leading experts in the fields of primary care, prevention, and evidence-based medicine. The USPSTF was created more than thirty years ago to provide primary care physicians with dependable recommendations on preventive medical services. What makes the USPSTF recommendations so dependable? Well, the USPSTF recommendations are "evidenced-based," which means that they are solely based on the current research available on any given preventive service. The USPSTF recommendations are also peer reviewed and publicly reviewed before publication. All of these measures ensure that the statements published by the USPSTF are the most authoritative, comprehensive recommendations of any given preventive services.[4]

In 2018, this task force published their official recommendations on prostate cancer screening. Based on their research, the USPSTF recommends that for men ages fifty-five to sixty-nine, prostate cancer screening should be an individual decision. They state that men should only make this decision after being fully informed of the potential benefits and harms of screening by their primary care physician. Age, family history, race/ethnicity, personal medical history, and individual preferences and values must all be considered before a final decision is made. Notably, for men over the age of seventy, the USPSTF does not recommend prostate cancer screening.[4]

In 2021, Richard M. Hoffman, MD, MPH, a graduate of Johns Hopkins University School of Medicine and current professor of internal medicine, echoed the findings of the USPSTF.[5] In his up-to-date review of the research on prostate cancer screening, Dr. Hoffman found that there is merit to screening, as it can have an impact on reducing metastatic prostate cancer cases and prostate cancer–related mortality. In addition to discussing the pros of screening, Dr. Hoffman also recognized the importance of identifying the cons of this preventive service. Therefore, in his paper he also explores the possible harmful effects of prostate cancer screening. These potential consequences can include anxiety, false positives, overdiagnosis, and the damage to quality of life that could result from prostate biopsies and/or treatment complications.[5] Due to these possible detriments and the generally slow progression of prostate cancer, Dr. Hoffman does not recommend that men with life expectancies of fewer than ten years undergo prostate cancer screening. Ultimately, like the USPSTF, Dr. Hoffman advocates for shared decision-making between men and their primary care physicians when it comes to prostate cancer screening.[5]

If after reading this chapter you still cannot decide if getting a PSA blood test is right for you, this would be an excellent opportunity to consult your primary care physician and see what they recommend based on your unique health profile.[4, 5] On the other hand, if you are now feeling motivated to discuss scheduling a PSA blood test with your physician, there are two more things you should know before proceeding.

First and foremost, you should know that there are two ways that PSA proteins can circulate in your bloodstream. Some PSAs circulate freely, while others travel attached to proteins in your blood.[3] Because there are two forms of the PSA protein that circulate in your bloodstream, scientists have created multiple PSA tests that analyze one or both of these PSA types. Each of the tests available today have their own strengths and weaknesses, but the purpose of them all remains the same: to determine your chances of currently having prostate cancer. Nowadays, your PSA screening blood test options are a total PSA test, a percent-free PSA test, and two varieties of combination PSA tests.[3]

1. Total PSA test: The most frequently used PSA screening is a total PSA blood test, which analyzes both forms of PSA in your bloodstream.[3]

2. Percent-free PSA test: This test creates a ratio only between the PSAs that are free (unattached to proteins) within your blood-

stream and the total amount of PSA in your blood. This test is useful because studies have found that men with prostate cancer have a lower percentage of free PSA when compared to men without prostate cancer. In other words, if you have a lower percentage of free PSA, you have a higher chance of having prostate cancer. The American Cancer Society recommendations suggest that if your percent-free PSA is lower than 10 percent, you should discuss having a prostate biopsy with your physician to determine if you have prostate cancer. If your percent-free PSA is between 10 and 25 percent, a prostate biopsy discussion is advised, especially if your total PSA is high as well.[3]

3. Combination PSA tests: While relatively new, combination PSA tests are another prostate cancer screening option. Combination PSA tests create an aggregated score based on your results from multiple PSA tests, which can be used to help find out the probability that you have prostate cancer and whether or not you should have a prostate biopsy. The two combination PSA tests available today are the prostate health index (combines total PSA, free PSA, and proPSA [premature form of PSA]) and the 4Kscore test (combines total PSA, free PSA, intact PSA, and human kallikrein 2).[3]

It is important to note that a high PSA test result does not automatically mean you have prostate cancer. There are many men with above-average PSA blood levels that do not have cancer. That said, if your PSA results are higher than normal, there are a few next steps you can take. The next step after an atypical PSA result will be different for each person, as it will depend on how high your PSA results are, your individual health profile (age, overall health, and personal risk for prostate cancer), and the discussions you have about this matter with your physician.

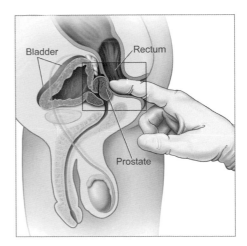

The digital rectal exam (DRE) is one of the most common follow-ups to an atypical PSA test, but it can also sometimes be conducted in tandem with the initial PSA test.[3] A DRE is a medical procedure that can help detect prostate cancer in men who either have normal PSAs or would like to follow up on a high PSA test result. The anatomical image on page 99, created by the National Cancer Institute, displays an in-process DRE.[6] During this procedure, the physician will insert a gloved finger into the rectum to feel if there are any abnormal bumps or hard spots on the prostate that could be cancerous. Oftentimes prostate cancer begins on the portion of the prostate that backs up to the rectum, so this fast exam, while uncomfortable, can be useful in identifying cancer in that region of the prostate.[3]

Aside from the DRE, if you have a high PSA result but no other risk factors for prostate cancer, you can consider waiting a few months and then completing a repeat PSA test. But, if you do have other risk factors, the American Cancer Society's guidelines suggest that further testing and/or a prostate biopsy might be the next best step for you. Further testing could come in the form of an MRI test of the prostate gland or a transrectal ultrasound (TRUS).[3] While these screening tests are informative, the only way to truly confirm if you have prostate cancer is through a diagnostic biopsy. During a prostate biopsy, a small piece of the prostate is removed and then analyzed under a microscope. This procedure can determine with certainty if a man has prostate cancer, and if he does, how quickly it will grow and spread.[3] As we've mentioned before, it is essential to discuss these advanced screening and diagnostic options with your primary care physician before making any decisions.

Routine Screening Options for Prostate Cancer

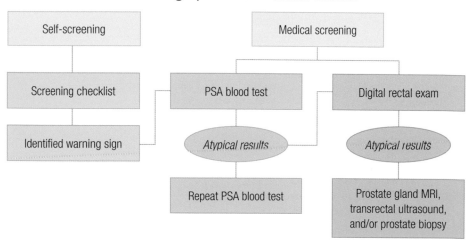

We have just reviewed a lot of different options for routine prostate cancer screening. If you are having difficulty keeping them all straight, don't worry—you are not alone.

To screen or not to screen? The answer to this dynamic question changes every year as new prostate screening tests are created and advancements are made in the world of prostate cancer research. Here's the bottom line: considering screening in one form or another is a critical aspect of prostate cancer prevention.[7] Adding a short, regular self-screening to your lifestyle is a simple choice, but before you begin scheduling some of the more advanced medical screening options it is important to know the risks and benefits of each test. Having an open and honest discussion with your physician can help you determine the appropriate next steps for your specific health profile.[7] This discussion will also give you the opportunity to ask yourself what your preferences and principles are when it comes to routine screening for prostate cancer. Ultimately, the best thing you can do is make a fully informed decision that both you and your physician agree is right for your prostate health.

BIBLIOGRAPHY CHAPTER 8

1. American Cancer Society (2010). Should I be tested for prostate cancer? *CA: A Cancer Journal for Clinicians*, 60(2):133. DOI:10.3322/caac.20062.

2. "Prostate Cancer Symptoms." Cancer Treatment Centers of America. December 2, 2021. www.cancercenter.com/cancer-types/prostate-cancer/symptoms.

3. American Cancer Society Medical and Editorial Content Team. "Screening Tests for Prostate Cancer." Accessed April 21, 2021. www.cancer.org/cancer/prostate-cancer/detection-diagnosis-staging/tests.html.

4. U.S. Preventive Services Task Force (2018). Screening for prostate cancer: U.S. Preventive Services Task Force recommendation statement. *JAMA*, 319(18):1901–1913. DOI:10.1001/jama.2018.3710.

5. Hoffman, R.M. (July 1, 2021). "Screening for Prostate Cancer." *UpToDate*. www.uptodate.com/contents/screening-for-prostate-cancer.

6. National Cancer Institute (2008). "Rectal Examination." National Cancer Institute. Accessed April 21, 2021. https://www.cancer.gov/types/prostate/patient/prostate-screening-pdq.

7. American Cancer Society Medical and Editorial Content Team. "American Cancer Society Recommendations for Prostate Cancer Early Detection." Accessed April 21, 2021. www.cancer.org/cancer/prostate-cancer/detection-diagnosis-staging/acs-recommendations.html.

Conclusion

L ifestyle and health are inextricably connected. Current research has found this to be true time and time again. You have just finished reviewing more than one hundred of the most valid articles on lifestyle factors and your risk of prostate cancer incidence. From your routine screening practices to your dietary and exercise choices, the decisions you make every day can determine the diseases you get and those you avoid. Hopefully this book has helped you realize how much power you have when it comes to your health, especially in relation to your risk of getting prostate cancer. The stories and research discussed in these eight chapters exist within the pages of this book; the next chapter of this narrative extends into real life, your life.

At this point, you may be feeling motivated to make some lifestyle changes. You may also be experiencing a little of motivation's best friend, uncertainty. Maybe you are uncertain about where to begin. Maybe you are uncertain about how to turn your new goals into actions, and those actions into habits. We've all made New Year's resolutions and then given up on them a month later, so how can you make these goals stick?

For starters, most New Year's resolutions are made about five minutes before the new year begins, with very little forethought. These goals are different. You have just dedicated yourself to reading an entire book with the sole purpose of informing yourself on these goals. You have reviewed data from a variety of studies on the topic of lifestyle choices and prostate cancer risk. Your takeaways from this book are not off-the-cuff resolutions; rather they are deeply educated decisions. However you choose to apply the information presented in this book, you know the choices you make will be made with conviction. If you choose to add a cup of broccoli to your dinner, it will be because you know that studies show that increasing your cruciferous vegetables intake may reduce your risk for getting prostate cancer. Let's be real—you'd be less likely to add that cup of broccoli if you were only doing it because someone else told you to. Goals that come from a place of knowledge are easier to stick to because they are made with conviction.

If you have decided to make an educated change to your lifestyle, start today and start small. By breaking up your goals into smaller chunks, they will become more achievable. Adding a twenty-minute walk to your day is a lot easier to stick with than forcing yourself to run for an hour every day. The more you complete the smaller activities, the easier they will become. Once the twenty-minute walk becomes routine, then you can build up to your next goal. The same is true for dietary changes. During the process of making health changes to your life, it is inevitable that you will make mistakes. Forgive yourself. You are not perfect and you shouldn't hold yourself to an unattainable standard. When forming healthier lifestyle habits, you should set a goal of continuous improvement. Understand that some days you will take steps forward and other days you will take steps back, and that is okay. Reflect regularly and improve continuously. Finally, accept that there is no right or wrong way to achieve your goals, only what works best for you.

You now have the tools to make lifestyle changes that can significantly impact your health. How you use these tools is up to you.

About the Authors

BENNY GAVI, MD, is a graduate of Harvard Medical School and current clinical assistant professor of medicine at Stanford University. For the first sixteen years of his career, Dr. Gavi practiced medicine in a hospital setting at Harvard and Stanford. In 2012, he expanded to an internal medicine practice to focus on personalized health care. In this position, Dr. Gavi has become a strong advocate for and expert on health improvement and disease prevention through nutrition and other life- 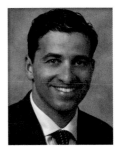 style factors. In addition to his medical practice, Dr. Gavi has spent the past decade sharing his passion for lifestyle choices and disease prevention through nutrition counseling and education.

MAYA EYLON is a Doctor of Medicine candidate at Central Michigan University College of Medicine, pursuing her passion for helping others through holistic health care and preventive medicine. She completed her Bachelor of Arts in Pre-Medicine Studies at Whittier College, and, as a clinical researcher interested in integrative lifestyle medicine, has conducted research with Hadassah Medical Center and Stanford University School of Medicine.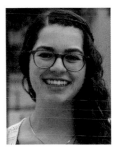

Index

Page references for figures are *italicized*.

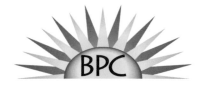

books that educate, inspire, and empower

To find your favorite books on plant-based cooking and nutrition, raw-foods cuisine, and healthy living, visit
BookPubCo.com.

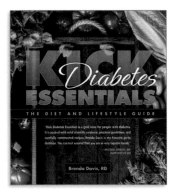

Kick Diabetes Essentials
The Diet and Lifestyle Guide
Brenda Davis, RD
978-1-57067-376-4 • $27.95

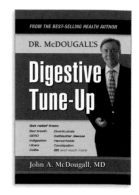

Dr. McDougall's
Digestive Tune-Up
John McDougall, MD
978-1-57067-184-5 • $19.95

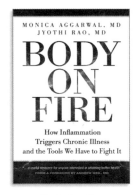

Body On Fire
How Inflammation Triggers Chronic Illness
and the Tools We Have to Fight It
Monica Aggarwal, MD and Jyothi Rao, MD
978-1-57067-392-4 • $17.95

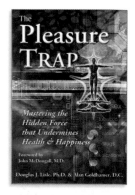

The Pleasure Trap
Mastering the Hidden Force That
Undermines Health & Happiness
Alan Goldhamer and Douglas J. Lisle
978-1-57067-197-5 • $16.95